BREAKING
THE
SILENCE

BREAKING THE SILENCE

Inspirational Stories of Black Cancer Survivors

KARIN L. STANFORD, Ph.D.

INTRODUCTION BY NIKKI GIOVANNI

HILTON PUBLISHING COMPANY • CHICAGO, ILLINOIS

Hilton Publishing Company
Chicago, IL

Direct all correspondence to:
Hilton Publishing Company
110 Ridge Road
Munster, IN 46321
815–885–1070
www.hiltonpub.com

Library of Congress Cataloging-in-Publication Data

Stanford, Karin L., 1961–
    Breaking the silence : inspirational stories of Black cancer survivors /
Karin L. Stanford.
        p. cm.
    Includes bibliographical references.
    ISBN 0-9716067-9-X (pbk. : alk. paper)
    1. Cancer—Patients—Biography. 2. African Americans—Diseases. I.
Title.
    RC265.5.S73 2005
    362.196'994'008996073—dc22   2005000558

Printed and bound in the United States of America

THIS BOOK IS DEDICATED TO THE SPECIAL PEOPLE IN MY
LIFE WHO HAVE BEEN TOUCHED BY CANCER: MYRTLE
(JOANN) GIBSON, TONI MONIQUE GRAYSON, ANDREA
HUNT, HEBRON HUNT, BEVERLY PORTER, CALVIN SMITH,
DAMU SMITH, AND KIMBERLY THORNE. AND, TO MY
FRIEND AND COMPANION, RONALD LEE JONES, WHOSE
VALIANT BALLTE WITH CANCER IS A TESTAMENT TO THE
STRENGTH OF THE SPIRIT. I CAN STILL HEAR YOU SINGING.

CONTENTS

Acknowledgments

This book is composed of many voices. The contributors shared not only their personal journeys with cancer, but also their friends', their children's, and other relatives' experiences. Their contributions are the heart and soul of this book. I thank them for their generosity of spirit and their willingness and desire to share their journey in order to help others.

Many others are responsible for turning the idea of this book into a reality. I depended upon a core group of friends and colleagues. Valerie C. Johnson, Ph.D., Ronald L. Jones, James Simmons, Esq., and Mary Thomas helped to transform this project from idea to book. They read drafts of the proposal, helped strategize on how to collect stories, and offered insights that shaped the end product. My two assistants Ana Thorne and Thandisizwe Chimerenga also provided strategic and logistical support. Thanks to Johnnie Scott and Tom Spencer-Walters, both professors at California State University, Northridge, who commented on the manuscript. A special thanks to Rick Blake, who helped to edit the manuscript, interview contributors, and provide professional comment on the overall project.

My love and thanks go to other friends who provided support and encouragement to me while I worked to complete this project. These friends not only gave their time to comment on this work, but also understood its emotional affect on me. Najee Ali, Mark Bush, Rafiki Cai, Maurice Carney, Edward Grice, Ronald Jones, and James Simmons, you are my champions. I hope that you will consider me a champion for you one day. Dori Bye, you picked up and carried the baton for the Black Cancer Network when I was busy working on this manuscript. You did so without question and without hesitation. You are greatly appreciated. Meri Danquah, thank you once for understanding my need to share my experience and thank you twice for helping me find the right words.

The women of the California Black Women's Health Project often clarified the importance of this work as a tool for helping black people advocate for themselves on important healthcare issues. Latonya Slack, Crystal Crawford, Trudi Butts, Holly Mitchell, and Karen Elliot Brown. I hope to live up to your example. Thank you for your insight and wisdom.

I want to thank my family and long-time friends for providing support, advice, and sometimes the basics, like lunch and dinner. Thank you for understanding the personal and emotional sacrifices it took to work on this subject. To my elders, Grandma Lucinda, Mom, Bobby, Pearl and Mel, Joann, Herbert and Pam, Hebron and Andrea, you have been my rock. To my sister, brother, and Wilma, thanks for entertaining Ashley as I slipped away to work. In addition to my family, my friends Joe Davidson, Cynthia Chase, Marlene Williams, Robyn Cook, Damu Smith, and Vanessa Hirsi supported me through my own treatment for breast cancer. Some of you flew thousands of miles to visit and care for me. Thank you, thank you. And finally to my nieces and nephews, thanks for giving Ashley and me joy.

I am also so very grateful to Michelle Jordan, my media consultant and friend. When others did, you refused to give up on me. You helped me regain my life and encouraged me to continue the work that I feel so passionate about.

To Hilton Publishing, thank you for taking the chance on this project. To my editors, Herbert Stern and Karla Dougherty, I appreciate your guidance, enthusiasm, and expertise. Elizabeth Gnatch, thank you for reading and editing, always at the last minute. I am so grateful for your support of all of my writing efforts.

I also had help from a generous group of physicians and specialists. My oncologist, Philomena McAndrew supported this project from the beginning. Thank you for taking time out of your busy schedule to contact others to help. You never neglected to inquire about the project and offer assistance. To Dr. Andrea Mitchell, an activist, physician and excellent practitioner, thank you for serving on the advisory board of the Black Cancer Network and reaching out to others on its behalf. Dr. Donald Henderson and Dr. Robert Dewitty also graciously agreed to serve on the BCN advisory committee and supported this work. You all are a great example to your profession. I am so pleased to have been blessed with your expertise.

To my support group, Rise Sister Rise in Washington D.C., you were the home for me when I had nowhere else to turn. I honor you. To Kimberly Thorne and others of Rise Sister Rise who made their transition, your spirit continues to strengthen us.

To Cynthia Oredugba and Hortensia Moore of the South Central Branch of the American Cancer Society, thanks so much for welcoming me into the family and for welcoming this work. You both exemplify caring and commitment.

A final and special thank you to my daughter, Ashley, for making me laugh and making me proud.

FOREWORD

I am searching for the language of cancer. I am not a victim; I have a disease. Though, with cancer, we always say we are fighting it; we will conquer it; we are overcoming. We *used* to have it.

I think we all always have cancer. Sometimes it shows itself; sometimes it doesn't. We have chemotherapy or we have surgery. Sometimes that works and a lot of time that doesn't. We use everything at our disposal. Sometimes we live; sometimes we die.

When I was diagnosed with lung cancer, I thought I would surely die. I had to take a moment to consider where I was. I was in that awkward position where I did not want to die but could find no reason to "pass this cup" to anyone else.

I prayed. I guess we all pray when cancer strikes. But I had a particular problem: I was not sure what to pray for. A longer life? Maybe . . . but at what cost? I prayed for grace. I just really didn't want to embarrass myself. I didn't want to whine. And I certainly didn't want to ask: Why me?

I thought about the men and women who, between 1892, the start of Black Laws, and 1955, the murder of Emmett Till, did not ask: Why Me? but who died bravely and with dignity to show how awful these people were among whom we lived. I thought of my ancestors who traveled over the Atlantic Ocean chained, whipped, branded and abused who did not ask, "Why Me? but who said: I will more than survive, I will live and thrive and sing a song so beautifully that the world will take notice of my humanity.

I wanted to be worthy.

Cancer is not a good neighbor nor a good friend. Yet it is not our enemy either. It is a disease that we must find a way to comfort and calm. We must find a way not to defeat it but to live with it. Like any bully, it must be called to order. But like any child on the schoolyard, it must be made to play fair.

I wish us luck. All of us will not be passed over. Those who are and those who aren't still must find a love that we can depend upon; still must lean on the everlasting arms.

There is a language of cancer. A language not of fear but of understanding, not of hatred but of love. When we change the way we look at cancer we may be able to change the way cancer looks at us. At any rate, it is a good idea to live. To notice early and to try to hold on to this most precious gift: our lives.

Nikki Giovanni
Poet/University Distinguished Professor
Virginia Polytechnic Institute and State University

THE FACT THAT WE ARE HERE AND THAT I SPEAK NOW
THESE WORDS IS AN ATTEMPT TO BREAK THAT
SILENCE AND BRIDGE SOME OF THOSE DIFFERENCES
BETWEEN US, FOR IT IS NOT DIFFERENCE WHICH
IMMOBILIZES US, BUT SILENCE. AND THERE ARE SO
MANY SILENCES TO BE BROKEN.

—Audre Lorde

IN ORDER TO HAVE A CONVERSATION WITH SOMEONE
YOU MUST REVEAL YOURSELF.

—James Baldwin, *Nobody Knows My Name*

Our Stories

CHAPTER ONE

My Personal Journey

Cancer. I listened as the words left my doctor's mouth. That single word traveled slowly through the air and settled in my ears. I decided, almost immediately, that it was improbable, that it had to be some sort of mistake, some sort of cruel joke. There was no way that I could have cancer. No way. Not me.

"Are you sure?" I asked. Thinking back on that day, it is the first question most people probably ask when they have just been told something devastating, life-altering, something utterly unbelievable. *Are you sure?*

I can only imagine that other people ask that same question for the same reasons that I asked it: they suddenly recognize the importance of that moment, the moment that has forever separated what has been from what will be. They want to go back in time and mark that moment clearly in their minds.

I know now that this is what I wanted, a way to provide a context for those words: *You have cancer.* I wanted to slow down and associate that revelation with something other than raw emotion, something concrete—the electric whiteness of the doctor's coat, the smooth cinnamon glow of his skin, the navy blue, double-breasted business suit I was wearing that day. Placed against the larger backdrop of my life, cancer made absolutely no sense to me. I was an African-American woman in my mid-thirties. I was practically a vegetarian; I exercised regularly; I didn't smoke; and was not aware of any family history of cancer. There was no way I could have cancer.

If I were going to truly understand the words the doctor had spoken, specifically what one word, cancer, meant to me, I was going to have to start with small, manageable details. *Are you sure?*

The question echoed in my mind, slowly, deliberately. Entire lifetimes passed in the time that I waited to hear my doctor's response. I saw my childhood, the fragrant smell of gingerbread in my grandmother's house and my youthful dreams, so many possibilities. But, mostly, I thought about the day that I first discovered that I had a lump in my breast.

It was 1997, around dinnertime and, as always, I was multi-tasking. My close girlfriend, Rachel, and I were talking on the phone while I was getting dressed to go to a reception, one of the many highbrow events to which I was invited in my role as bureau chief of the Washington, D.C., Office of the RainbowPUSH Coalition. It was a typical conversation, girlfriend gossip. Rachel was catching me up on the madness that our mutual friend was being subjected to by her boyfriend.

I had opened up a package of Hanes™ stockings and removed the sheer, gentle brown pantyhose from the cardboard insert around which it had been wrapped. As I was about to toss the insert into the trash, I noticed that there was some writing on the back of it. I looked closer and saw that it was a set of instructions on how to do a self-breast examination. Had I been in more of a hurry, I might have just thrown the insert away without taking another look. I would have never known or even wondered about the message that the people at Hanes had hoped their consumers would read.

This time, I was easing myself into the evening. I wanted to arrive at the reception late, fashionably so. I sat down at the foot of my bed, dropped the pantyhose beside me, and, while still talking to Rachel, proceeded to read the insert and then do the step-by-step exam. I didn't think anything of it—just a mindless activity, something to do with my hands while I was chitchatting on the phone.

I felt a lump. Shocked, I returned my fingers back to that spot and caressed it again. Rachel was still talking. I shifted my attention from the conversation to the cardboard insert and reread the instructions. I repeated the exam on the same breast. Again, I felt the lump. A feeling of concern, more than fear, hit me. I interrupted Rachel to tell her I'd just done a breast self-exam and had found a lump. "Girl, don't even trip," she said, dismissing my concern in that lovingly casual way our friends use to sweep away our many irrational and unfounded worries. "It's probably nothing but a cyst, if even that. Just go to the doctor and have it removed."

Rachel knew a lot about cysts because she was constantly discovering them on various parts of her body. She'd undergone several minor surgeries to have them removed. There was wisdom in what she was telling me.

When I went to the gynecologist, he did what I had already done, a breast exam, and told me what I already knew–that there was a lump in my breast and that it was probably a cyst. He advised me to wait and see what happened. Being a researcher by training, I knew that facts were always better than educated guesses. I instinctively knew not to trust the "wait and see" attitude, especially not when it came to my health; I wanted *definitely*. I wanted, and asked for, a mammogram. The gynecologist thought it was unnecessary and, at first, he refused to give me a referral. But I was insistent. I needed to know exactly what that lump was.

I pleaded with the doctor and two months later—an ultrasound and a needle biopsy later—I finally got those definitive results. I was sitting in a doctor's office at Howard University Hospital in Washington, D.C. It was in the middle of a workday and I was in my business attire, briefcase in hand—all the symbols of my hard-earned success. It was there that I watched my dreams dissolve. I felt myself fade into my surroundings.

Are you sure?

By the time the doctor spoke, I had already retreated into a place of safety—Without a pause, I'd stepped over the threshold and entered a world of fantasy. When he said, "Yes, Karin, I am sure," it was not his voice I heard; it was my mother's, my aunts' and grandmother's. And it was not a confirmation of illness but an affirmation of life. It came to me as a challenge. And I dared to believe that I would prevail.

Fast-forward to Friday, June 18, 1999. One morning, a year and a half later, I stormed into the office of my oncologist, looked him straight in the eye, and asked, "Should I cut off my breasts to save my life?" He gazed back at me, as if assessing my mood and trying to discover with his eyes what had prompted that question.

Less than a month before, I had given birth to my only child, Ashley. It was supposed to be a joyous time. Despite the advice of several physicians that I should have strongly considered terminating my pregnancy, I took a leap of faith. So, even after chemotherapy, radiation, and seemingly limitless medication to manage the side effects from the cancer treatment, the pregnancy went extremely well. Ashley had been born healthy and I had not experienced any major complications.

My physicians feared that my pregnancy might trigger a breast cancer recurrence. Eight months after treatment for Stage IIA Infiltrating Ductal Carcinoma, I discovered that I was pregnant. My oncologist explained to me that there was very little scientific data on pregnancy and cancer, especially in African-American women. I would become a guinea pig of sorts for my physicians and others.

Even though Ashley was born healthy, and I was declared healthy after her birth, I was terribly afraid. Here she was, a helpless, defenseless baby, who might not have a mom to care for her. Perhaps I had risked my life so that she would be born, but maybe it would come at too high a price for both of us. I was willing to do whatever it took to reduce the chances of a recurrence of cancer.

My oncologist warned me that all surgeries have risks and that there are no guarantees; even drastic measures, such as undergoing a preventative double mastectomy, might not work. He wanted to monitor my progress and take a methodical approach to my illness. Eight years and several physicians later, I am still here.

My Cancer Education

Since my diagnosis in January 1997, I have become a connoisseur of cancer-related material. I've read literature from medical textbooks, books about herbal remedies and prevention, as well as memoirs written by others who have had cancer. I can now describe the facts about cancer deftly, as if they don't even frighten me. Examining the raw facts head on is an important step forward.

The term cancer refers to the out-of-control growth of damaged cells. Healthy cells grow and divide to produce additional cells, as the body needs them. Cancer cells grow, divide, and form more cells when the body does not need them. These extra cells typically form a mass of tissue called a tumor. All tumors, however, are not cancerous. A cancerous tumor is malignant, and a non-cancerous tumor is benign and rarely life threatening.[1]

Some cancer cells, resulting in cancers such as leukemia and lymphoma, do not form tumors but arise in the blood and blood-forming organs and circulate through other tissue. However, these types of cancers can invade other organs and can form tumors there.

There are over thirty-five types of cancer, most of them named for the organ or type of cell in which they begin. Metastasis occurs when cancer cells travel away from the original site to other parts of the body and begin to grow, replacing normal tissue. When cancer metastasizes, cancer cells typically find their way into lymph nodes and lymph glands.

Although it is the second leading cause of death in the United States, cancer can be treated. The American Cancer Society estimates that more than 550,000 Americans—or more than 1,500 people a day—die of cancer every year.[2]

Cancer does not affect all races equally. For instance, cervical cancer incidence is two to three times higher among Mexican and

---

1. American Cancer Society, *Detailed Guide: What Is Cancer?* (2003), <www.cancer.org>; George Rawls, Frank P. Lloyd Jr., and Herbert Stern, *Managing Cancer: The African American's Guide to Prevention, Diagnosis, and Treatment* (Roscoe, Ill.: Hilton Publishing, 2001), 13–14.
2. American Cancer Society, *Cancer Facts and Figures* (Atlanta: The Society, 2004).

Puerto Rican women than in non-Hispanic White women. Vietnamese men have the highest rates of liver cancer for all racial/ethnic groups.[3] There are also age and gender differences. Cancer will most likely strike older people.

Cancer is treated by a combination of surgery, chemotherapy, radiation, and a host of alternative therapies. The type of cancer and whether or not it has spread from the original site are the two most critical factors in determining treatment. Medical history can also factor into treatment decisions.

Despite the grim statistics of the past, cancer survival rates are improving, and cancer patients are living longer—and even beating the disease.[4] Not only are those stricken with the disease surviving, but they are experiencing a better quality of life while undergoing treatment. Today, surgery is less radical, chemotherapy is producing fewer side effects and new medications have been developed to combat the difficult side effects of treatment. Survival rates also vary by cancer types, the stage of diagnosis and one's age upon diagnosis. To this extent, survival rates are typically discussed in relative terms and will vary based on individual circumstances.

My understanding of the unique African-American experience with cancer first occurred when I set out to locate a support group. I attended a support group meeting of one well-known cancer-focused organization but could not identify with the women in the group. Most of them were White, over fifty, and

---

3. Intercultural Cancer Council, Fact Sheets, Hispanics/Latinos & Americans and Cancer, Fact Sheets, Asian Americans and Cancer.
4. American Cancer Society, Facts and Figures, 2004.

had children. I was relatively young, single, and African American. In addition to the demographic differences, I soon discovered that my prognosis was different. Because I am an African-American female, my chances for survival were less than those of my White counterparts. Armed with this information, I began to search for support organizations that would be more compatible. Through research and with the help of my surgeon, I found a very supportive and spiritually uplifting group, "Rise Sister Rise,"* whose members were all African-American women battling breast cancer. These women, or might I say, "these sistas," understood my circumstances from the moment I walked in the door. They challenged me to "rise." With the help of this support group, I learned about prevention, treatment, and how to cope with the disease. I also learned that in spite of our diagnoses, we could still live and live well.

As a result of my involvement with Rise Sister Rise, I became educated about how race and ethnicity can factor into a cancer diagnosis. It's hard enough when a person finds out she has cancer and has to deal with that devastating information—but to then have to contend with receiving inferior care? That's not true in every instance, but too often inadequate health insurance, racial insensitivity and unequal medical treatment create additional burdens for people of color facing cancer.

---

* The Rise Sister Rise! Support Group is a program of the Breast Cancer Resource Committee. For more information, go to <www.aframerica.com/bcrc>. Also see the Resource Guide for additional information on Rise Sister Rise! and other support groups in your local area.

Within the African-American community approximately 130,800 new cases of cancer are diagnosed annually.[6] Among African-American women, breast, colon and rectal, lung, cervical, and uterine cancer are most prevalent. For African-American men, prostate, lung, colon and rectal, non-Hodgkin's lymphoma, and stomach cancer are more likely.[7]

Disparities in cancer incidence, survival, and mortality illustrate that the disease disproportionately disrupts African-American lives. African Americans have the highest death rate from all cancers combined and survival rates are shorter for African Americans than Whites at all stages of diagnosis.[8] These differences have been associated with higher poverty among African Americans, reduced access to medical care, increased environmental risks, and late diagnoses. African Americans also tend to make less use of screening and early detection procedures than Whites in this country.

This may be, in part, associated with racism in the health care industry, but it may also result from African-Americans' long-standing mistrust of the medical profession and their failure to discuss cancer openly. Yet, despite these harsh statistics, there has been improvement in the African-American 5-year survival rates, the benchmark used in most studies. From 1960 through 1963, the survival rate for African Americans afflicted with cancer was 27 percent, compared to 49 percent during the 1989–96 period.[9]

---

6. Intercultural Cancer Council, *Fact Sheets: African Americans and Cancer* (2001).
7. From Selected Data Sources, including Managing Cancer, American Cancer Society, National Cancer Institutes.
8. American Cancer Society, *Cancer Facts and Figures;* Intercultural Cancer Council, *Fact Sheets.*
9. American Cancer Society, "Cancer Fact and Figures for African-Americans."

BLACK CANCER MYTHS

In my quest to understand the African-American cancer experience, I found that very few of us had spoken publicly about the illness. Even more notable was that a diagnosis of cancer within the African-American community carried a particular stigma. Many African Americans considered having cancer shameful and would therefore not admit to having the disease— or even to having a close relative that suffers from it. Despite its prevalence, many people still refer to cancer quietly as the "Big C."

Myths abound around cancer within the African-American community, and, in my conversations with African Americans about my own diagnosis, I uncovered five that most commonly permeate our response to cancer.

Myth Number One: African Americans rarely get cancer.

I, myself, had subscribed to this belief. So when I found a lump in my breast, it never occurred to me, my gynecologist, or my close friends and family members that I, in fact, had cancer. Even my own doctor had encouraged me to take a "wait-and-see" approach. Unfortunately, such thinking can lead to a late diagnosis and, ultimately, fewer treatment options.

Myth Number Two: Cancer is always fatal.

The fatalistic belief that cancer is incurable leads to a fear of diagnosis and, therefore, later detection becomes more likely. Yet, more than 50 percent of cancers can be successfully treated, and for some cancers, the success rate is very high. Unfortunately, among African Americans, cancer is frequently diagnosed after the cancer has metastasized and spread to regional or distant sites. This makes beating the disease much more difficult.

Since cancer is more likely to be treated successfully if it's detected early, regular check-ups are crucial. Having frequent cancer screenings and seeing a doctor as soon as you exhibit symptoms can also lead to earlier detection. Although cancer detection is not an easy subject to embrace, understanding more about the disease helps remove some of the fear and gives us the tools we need to prevent it.

Myth Number Three: Surgery will cause the cancer to spread.

A common refrain within the African-American community—"I am not going to let those doctors cut on me"—reflects a deep mistrust of physicians. A friend of mine bragged about his mother's refusal to have surgery for a bleeding lump found in her breast. He told me that his mother, who worked in a hospital, knew about the mistakes that doctors make during surgical procedures. My friend's mother passed away a year later.

This mistrust is reflective of the injustices that African Americans have previously suffered from the medical establishment. One example is the widely known Tuskegee Experiment, a 40-year, government funded study where African-American men were deliberately left to suffer and deteriorate from syphilis. Other horror stories include the forced sterilization of African-American women on welfare throughout the country.

The idea that surgery will cause the cancer to spread is also reflective of the historical mistrust that many African Americans feel toward the medical community. This belief has its roots in the days before we had adequate screening technology, which meant that a majority of patients already had very advanced cancers by the time they sought medical care. Frequently, doctors performed surgery to find the cause of a patient's illness; during the operation, they would find cancer that was too far advanced for successful treatment. When the patient died a short time later, observers thought the surgery had caused the cancer cells to spread—which led to the patient's death.

To combat these misunderstandings about cancer and its treatment, African Americans must be informed that, in many cases, surgery is, in fact, an essential aspect of cancer treatment. Surgery is frequently used to remove a cancerous tumor and nearby tissues that might contain cancer cells. Specialists in cancer surgery know how to take biopsy samples safely and to remove tumors without causing the cancer to spread. Doctors who perform surgery for cancer are specialists who have been trained to deal with the intricacies of cancer and anatomy. If patients or their families are concerned about their doctor's qualifications to perform surgery, they can contact the American Board of Medical Specialties, which certifies and evaluates physicians, or the American Medical Association's Physicians Select Program, which provides information on virtually every licensed physician in the United States.

Myth Number Four: Cancer is contagious.

Some people worry that they can catch cancer from other people, especially if the cancer is around the genital area (e.g., cervical cancer in women or testicular or prostate cancer in men). Despite such worries, cancer isn't a disease that can be transmitted to other people.

Myth Number Five: Cancer is a punishment for something a person has done wrong.

More than any other, this myth has probably enhanced the stigma associated with cancer. I have had to bite my tongue when friends or even strangers suggested that my cancer diagnosis was the result of "God trying to get my attention" because of some past mistake. Others had claimed that I had gotten cancer because I "snacked too much" or ate microwaved food. This way of thinking puts the blame for having cancer squarely on the patient. Certainly, it would have been tempting to answer, "Well, since we are all sinners, what do you think God's going to give you, and why is he waiting so long?" In my research, cancer survivors told me again and again that others had blamed their lifestyle or emotional instability or lack of attending church for their cancer.

The "blame game" makes many African-American cancer patients shy away from discussing their diagnosis openly; they fear that others will blame them for getting the disease. Accepting the myth that we have caused our cancers has dangerous repercussions. It can lead to a late diagnosis, as well as discourage people from thinking, reading, and writing about or openly discussing the disease. Sadly, it may also compel those who are experiencing the emotional trauma related to a cancer diagnosis to remain silent.

In my search for information about African Americans' experiences with cancer, I quickly discovered that other survivors have been searching, too. We talked among ourselves and as a result of these conversations we uncovered even more questions. Some of our questions concerned the medical and treatment aspects of cancer, but others involved the human side of being an African American with cancer.

We knew that there were support groups for those diagnosed with breast cancer, but were unsure about the existence of organized groups for African Americans afflicted with prostate, stomach, or lung cancer. What is the quality of life for African Americans after treatment? How are African Americans coping with the fear of recurrence? What about children with cancer and caregivers of cancer patients? What has led to the silence about cancer within the African-American community? How do we end the silence so that we can better educate our community on how to fight this disease? How do we give a voice to those who have had cancer and how do we validate that experience as worthy of open dialogue and discussion? The answers to these questions are complex and evolving and deserve to be shared with others who are concerned about African American's cancer experiences.

THE BIRTH OF BREAKING THE SILENCE

After deciding to write a book about African-American cancer survivors my close friends, colleagues, and family members worked with me to craft a "request for letters." We sent out countless requests via e-mail, phone and fax as well as press releases. We did not receive an overwhelming response from survivors. At first the letters came in slowly, cautiously. Nonetheless, the supporters of this project were determined that it would succeed, so they amplified their involvement with personal calls, letters, and e-mails to their friends, family, colleagues, and others who had experienced cancer. They asked their friends to tell other friends about the project, all in an attempt to collect more letters and stories.

I knew that it was important to hear from people from all walks of life, with many different stories. To that end, potential contributors were asked to respond to several questions. The questions ranged from the nature of their diagnosis to what the reaction was from family members and friends, and how they dealt with the changes in their physical appearances and emotions.

Some of the survivors replied right away. Others had a burning desire to tell their stories, but they did not believe they possessed adequate writing skills. We worked with them to help craft their narratives. There was also a special group of contributors who had become activists to support African Americans with cancer, some of whom wanted very much to share their experiences, but in their case, did not have adequate time to write. In those instances, they dictated their stories and we transcribed their tapes. We also recorded the stories of those at the end of life who could no longer write, but who wanted to contribute to the book. This book is the end product of all these efforts.

The contributors to *Breaking the Silence* range from individuals who are newly diagnosed to those who had completed treatment, to long-term survivors. Caregivers and family members shared their own experiences as well as the experiences of their loved ones who have made their transition. The contributors discuss their emotions: shock, grief, fear, laughter, and faith to a renewed appreciation of life. Through these letters we learn about some "universals" of the cancer experience that cut across divisions of race, class, and education. But we also learn how African Americans, in particular, cope with a cancer diagnosis.

This book is organized around important issues African–American cancer survivors must cope with. For example:

- the moment when the diagnosis is first learned
- the process of choosing the best treatment options
- the decision to start treatment—and when
- the role of race in cancer issues
- the effort to heal from cancer mentally, emotionally, and physically

- the reasons survivors became cancer awareness activists—
  and how

The stories are presented here in letter form; most of them address more than one issue, so the categories are flexible. The stories you will read here are too human to be confined to any one fixed "category" or issue. For example, you'll meet a number of African Americans whose faith carried them through the process of diagnosis, treatment, and healing, and who, once they were healed, became activists.

The cancer survivors who contributed letters to this project vary by age, sex, geographic location, and life experiences. The types of cancer treatment regiment also vary. The contributors reflect the range of demographics and personalities that exist within the African-American community. Some contributors refused conventional treatments, preferring instead to accept alternative therapies; others confronted cancer while incarcerated, while some, like me, are single parents, struggling to survive in order to raise young children. Although different, by recounting their own experiences, the survivors share a common goal: to provide assistance to those who are battling the illness. They also seek to promote messages about early detection, the importance of treatment, and emotional recovery. And, by putting their experiences into words, these survivors want their experiences to be shared. They hope to put an end to the silence that surrounds this disease.

My own belief is that in order to reduce pain and suffering and even save lives in the African-American community, we must recognize our own mistaken mythologies surrounding this disease. We must fight for equal access to medical care, adequate health insurance and more research on the environmental causes of cancer. In this way, we as a nation and as a people can change the dire statistics that still threaten the lives of so many.

* * * *

Cancer has a way of changing the course of one's life. Had it not been for cancer, for the fact that I thought I might die in my thirties, I might not have taken the opportunity to consider my life, to examine its purpose and to explore its possibilities.

Everyone, as the saying goes, has a story to tell. Until recently, I didn't think that mine was extraordinary. Now, like the contributors to this book, I am convinced that all of our stories are worth sharing and worth hearing. They are stories that we are not dying to tell. Instead, these are written testaments to what we have lived through, despite all odds.

CHAPTER TWO

Diagnosis

ONE'S OWN STRUGGLE IS INDIVIDUAL, BUT IT IS NOT
UNIQUE. ALL OF LIFE IS INVOLVED; STRUGGLE IS AN
INESCAPABLE ASPECT OF LIFE ITSELF.

—Howard Thurman, *Mediations of the Heart*

Ericka

Like many African Americans, Ericka couldn't find time to go in for a check-up. Her treatment was difficult, but it made her see that we are all "united by our determination and a resilient spirit."

My Love Diagnosis

In September of 1998, at the age of 27, I began to experience the early warning signs of cancer. I was a dental assistant and had been working in a new job for about one month when I began to feel really cold. I mentioned to my co-worker that it was freezing cold in the office. She replied, "The air conditioner isn't on. I think you are probably coming down with the flu." So I put a sweater over my scrub uniform. The following day, the temperature in the office felt the same. I was trembling and my teeth were chattering. Eventually, I laid my head down on the table. By then I knew that something was wrong. My office manager suggested that I go home early, but I was apprehensive because I was a new employee. She assured me that I could leave. I left thinking, "What if I can't return to work soon? Will my employer hire someone else in my place?"

My symptoms included shortness of breath, persistent chest pains, heart palpitations, weight loss, and night sweats. I took Tylenol 3 to relieve the pain in my chest. I eventually discovered an unusually large lump near my collarbone. I had gone from a healthy 135 pounds to a size four. Friends and family members began to notice the changes in me and asked if I had been dieting. I became self-conscious and wanted desperately to regain my weight because I was beginning to look sick.

I hesitated to seek medical attention. I had no medical benefits because I had not passed my probationary period at my new job. Plus, I was focused on my new career. I was in the process of continuing my education, studying to take the California State Board Exam to obtain R.D.A. (registered dental assistant certification). My long-term goal was to become a dental hygienist.

My mother pleaded with me to see a doctor. So I went to a free clinic, where I met Cheryl, a wonderful nurse. Cheryl was a devout Muslim who helped me relax while she examined me and took blood tests. That evening, she called and said that my blood count was abnormal. She urged me to pick up the lab results and go straight to the emergency room. My father drove me to pick up the report and then to the hospital.

I was told that I had Hodgkin's Disease, but not to worry, because it was a "good cancer." I whispered under my breath, "No, she didn't say that." I did not know that any cancer could be good. I had thought at worst that I had pneumonia. I followed up with an oncologist the next day and I prayed that God would protect me.

I knew that this was a spiritual test. It was also a test of emotional and physical endurance. I believed God had a plan for my life. "'For I know the plans I have for you,' declares the Lord, 'plans to prosper you and not to harm you, plans to give you hope and a future.'" (Jeremiah 29:11) I read these scriptures daily to cope when I got depressed. Another scripture that was important to me was, "And we know that in all things God works for the good of those who love him." (Romans 8:28) The news about my diagnosis traveled. I was blessed with the support of friends and family members.

I was told that because I was diagnosed in the early stages, my prognosis was good. I was thankful. After meeting with my doctor at Martin Luther King Drew Medical Center in Los Angeles, I chose conventional treatment, which included chemotherapy. After one year of successful treatment, I went into remission. However, six months later, I experienced a relapse. My doctor informed me that there was nothing else he could do for me. While he spoke, the tears streamed down my face. I was devastated. My doctor referred me to the City of Hope National Medical Center in Duarte, California, for a second opinion. Dr. Arif Alam from the Department of Hematology and Bone Marrow Transplantation reviewed my tests and X-rays. After the review he told me that I was eligible for a bone marrow transplant (BMT).

My stress level rose. I had applied for medical insurance several months earlier and was denied. Miraculously, my previous doctor and social worker helped me to obtain insurance so I was able to have the procedure. I immediately began pre-admission tests and a painful bone marrow biopsy. This procedure is very important because it helps determine bone marrow function.

I had an autologous transplant, which means "from yourself." It requires the removal or harvesting of some of your own healthy bone marrow or stem cells. The bone marrow is frozen and stored, then given back intravenously with a combination of high-dose chemotherapy and full-body radiation. I stayed in the hospital for two months. The most grueling part of the BMT was the high-dose chemotherapy. The transplant was successful, but I still have an inoperable tumor. It is next to my heart, which makes surgery risky. However, the tumor is non-viable, meaning that it is not growing. I am grateful for this second chance at life. It has been six years and I am now thirty-three years old!

Believe it or not, my name for chemo is "love juice." It is God's love and healing power working through the medicine that has helped me stay alive. Every day that I'm blessed to wake up is my birthday. Life is to be celebrated—it's a precious gift.

I believe none of us are strangers in this world. Throughout my cancer journey, I have met so many incredible people in the cancer community. We are united by our determination and resilient spirits. I am now a volunteer for the Los Angeles Chapter of the Leukemia Lymphoma Society. My work is focused on advocacy and fundraising for research. When I am not working with the society, I give free manicures and pedicures to cancer survivors and their caregivers.

I dedicate this letter to my loving family and friends and especially to my mother for her love, patience, and endurance as a caregiver and an inspiration. This letter is also dedicated to my brothers and sisters who are on the frontlines of the cancer war with me. I'm proud to be a fellow survivor.

ERICKA WALKER

Jerome

Jerome was comforted by the belief that he'd never need a marrow transplant. He thought he knew what a dreadful business the donor and donee might go through before, during, and after the procedure. Then he found out that he needs a transplant and that donors would be hard to find, since few African Americans donate marrow. Jerome thinks we should all educate ourselves about the procedure and about how to become donors.

A few years ago, I saw a newscast about a famous baseball player's daughter who had been diagnosed with leukemia. She was having a difficult time finding a bone marrow donor because she had a rare form of the disease and because her ethnic background was "mixed." I knew that she was fighting for her life and I remember my heart going out to her. I also remember not knowing anything about the process for donating bone marrow. I thought the doctor extracted the marrow from the donor's spine, and that no one would volunteer for such a painful procedure. Ignorance isn't always bliss.

Then, around October 2002, I began to lose my appetite and some of my athletic abilities. I literally had no stamina when exercising. After complaining to my doctor about a strange feeling in my stomach and the fact that I was tiring out too quickly, I was diagnosed with anemia. Shortly thereafter, a co-worker mentioned that she had acid reflux. A few months later, I ran into an old high school girlfriend whom I at first wanted to avoid. Without my prompting, she began to talk about having acid reflux during her pregnancy some ten years earlier. I talked to my son about my belief that I might have acid reflux and we agreed that it could become serious. So my son urged me to go to the emergency room.

When the emergency room doctor thanked me for coming in and insisted that I not leave, I wondered, "Since when does a doctor thank a patient for coming in?" After some tests, she explained to me that my white blood cell counts had gone through the roof. She also said that I might have leukemia and that they needed to admit me right away.

On February 11, 2003, at the age of thirty-eight, I was diagnosed with chronic myeloid leukemia or CML. I later found out that if I had waited another month to see a doctor I would not have lived. It was ironic! I thought that no one in my family had experienced cancer. I'd always been told that diabetes ran in my family, but not cancer. I learned that my assumptions weren't true. It turns out my grandfather lived with prostate cancer for ten years. He just passed early this year from complications with his kidneys. I also discovered that cancer killed most of his siblings.

As African Americans, we are not immune to cancer. We should educate ourselves about various forms of it and how we're affected. Out of necessity, I have learned a lot about donating bone marrow. I am now currently in need of a bone marrow transplant, and therefore contacting relatives to see who may be a match for me. I know that finding a match will be difficult. One reason is that I am the only child of my mother and father, although I have several half-siblings. In addition, I am of mixed race ancestry, which includes a mixture of African American, Native American, and French. I have just recently discovered that the best match for me is someone of Caribbean or Black and Hispanic heritage.

Marrow transplants are important to my survival because these transplants are the most effective way to treat my kind of leukemia, and other cancers too. To our detriment, we African Americans are not informed or proactive on the issue of donating marrow or organs. But here is what I have learned. For the donor, donating bone marrow is a simple 30 minute procedure that is practically pain-free when performed by a skilled doctor. Oh, and the marrow is extracted from just below the hip. There is a risk, but only to the patient receiving the marrow, not to the donor. Cancer patients receiving the marrow believe that a second chance at life is well worth the risk.

It has been one and a half years since I was diagnosed. In that time, I have come to realize that cancer plagues us all—from the patient to family members, caregivers, and friends. And yet, God does work in mysterious ways. From the very beginning, I knew God had it under control. He sent His angels to watch over me— including my ex-girlfriend, a co-worker, my son and daughter—even before my diagnosis. I don't believe in coincidence. God was trying to tell me something: Get to the hospital! Going through treatment, I knew His angels were everywhere. Through the medical staff at the hospital, and by way of neighbors, friends, cancer help-lines and total strangers, He had my back.

It's funny. While I was going through treatment, my doctor asked me why I didn't seem the least bit concerned about having this disease. A nurse told me, "God gave you this disease 'cause He knew you could handle it."

That's not to say that it's been blissful. As I've shared my dilemma with others, I've watched friends fall by-the-wayside. Girlfriends who once said that they loved me eventually abandoned me. I've realized that not everyone is capable of handling my situation. And yet, in some respects, I still view this disease as a blessing and not a curse. It was my wake-up call, because I was not living my life to the fullest. Now I am, although I can't say I don't have my bad days.

My doctors decided to put me on a new medication which scientists consider to be one of the new miracle drugs for cancer.

Within six months of taking it, the disease was almost eliminated from my system. The doctors even thought I might have been successfully treated. But I was not and it was devastating. My dosage was later increased but my body could not withstand the higher amount. Within a few short weeks, I was hospitalized with virtually no immune system. And now I need a bone marrow transplant.

Yes, I have had my moments of doubt. During those times, I felt like my mind, body, and soul had given up. Then a friend told me that her sister said she needs to check in on Jerome. She prayed that God would strengthen my body and spirit. And for my part, the thought of my daughter and son, whom I love dearly, growing up without me is unbearable. I need to claim and defeat this disease in the name of Jesus.

As my preacher father would say, "God is good, His mercy is everlasting, and His truth endures through all generations."

JEROME GREGORY WILLIAMS

William

For William, the cancer diagnosis was a kind of double indemnity. Seven years ago he had a quadruple heart bypass. After he had lived through an operation that removed 13 inches of his colon and endured 51 weeks of chemotherapy, William no longer was part of the "Thank God It's Friday" chorus. His anthem had become "Thank God It's Another Friday," because every day is precious to him.

I was diagnosed with colon cancer in February of 2000, at the age of 59.

It all began in September of 1999. After sweeping the kitchen floor, I found myself extremely tired. Ascending the stairs to the bedroom left me exhausted. In addition to the exhaustion, I suffered with severe constipation. In March of 1992, I had had quadruple heart bypass surgery and I assumed that I was having heart trouble again. But the cardiologist determined that my heart was not the problem.

Because the fatigue continued, I went to see my family doctor for a complete physical. He found that my blood count was extremely low and that I had blood in my stool. He had two units of blood administered to me and immediately I felt as good as new (I'm assuming this is how a drug addict feels after receiving a fix.) Nonetheless, the doctor wanted to know why I was losing blood, so he had me visit a gastroenterologist for a colonoscopy. The gastroenterologist discovered that I had polyps that had developed into cancer, penetrating through the wall of my colon. Surgery was necessary.

Thirteen inches of my colon were removed. The surgeon suggested that I take a year of chemotherapy to kill any cancer cells that may have moved to the lymph nodes. A port was surgically implanted just below my collarbone to administer the chemotherapy.

I was fortunate. The chemotherapy that I received for my type of colorectal cancer did not cause hair loss and through 51 weekly treatments I only had one minor bout with nausea. My only real side effects were dry and darkened hands and feet, which cleared up about three months after the chemotherapy was completed.

I now have a colonoscopy, a CT scan and an ultrasound annually, in addition to my routine doctor visits and, to date, all is well. When I hear my co-workers say after a trying week on the job, "Thank God It's Friday," I quietly say to myself, after undergoing two major surgeries, "Thank God for *another* Friday."

WILLIAM L. MCGRAW

Beverly

When Beverly was diagnosed, she became a warrior. Sick and tired of uncaring and unprofessional treatment from her HMO doctors, she stormed out of two doctors' offices and took charge of her health. Today, she sees her ordeal as the seed of her courage. Not only did she survive, but, by telling her story, she is helping others.

After I was told that I might have breast cancer, these were the questions I asked:

"What do you mean, another mammogram?"

"How can you perform a biopsy without seeing my X-rays and my file?"

"How can you give me a second opinion without seeing my X-rays?"

"What does HMO stand for? 'How Many Others?'"

But before I could ask these questions, I was in full denial. To myself I wondered how this could be; there was no history of breast cancer in my family. I felt as though I had been sucker-punched in the gut and was reeling from the blow. It was hard enough dealing with such devastating news, but soon my path would also be cluttered with horrible experiences with doctors and medical insurance. Sometimes in the midst of battle I wondered why everything was going so wrong. I now look back at my journey as the best thing that could have happened to me.

It all began when I went in for a second mammogram on September 25, 1996. My follow-up appointment two weeks later to discuss my X-rays with the surgeon was a total waste of time. The doctor had not seen the X-rays at all and ended up giving me some off-the-cuff, haphazard information that had been relayed to him by a radiologist over the phone.

The surgeon said that he would take a look at the X-rays and, if I wasn't contacted within a week, I should go ahead and schedule an appointment for a biopsy. Of course, I heard from no one, so I scheduled the biopsy appointment accordingly. Guess what? I was on the operating table and prepped when the surgeon finally looked at the X-rays just before entering the room. He determined that a biopsy was not possible because there were too many calcifications in my left breast! You don't say!

This sloppy treatment made me very nervous and doubtful; I wanted to get a second opinion. My primary physician requested that I go to a breast center via my HMO; the request was denied. I ended up seeing another doctor within the HMO. Silly me, I had high hopes. But the second doctor was no better than the first. As he was asking me questions about what the first doctor had told me, I realized that he hadn't seen my file or my X-rays either. I called him on it and he confessed and immediately put the blame on his staff. I had had more than enough; I stormed out of the office in a rage.

My anger gave me the energy to fight. It seemed as though the cancer had become secondary; my main focus was on dealing with the red tape strung up by the medical and insurance establishments to keep me from getting proper treatment.

I immediately faxed a letter to my insurance company describing the unprofessional and uncaring treatment I had received and demanded that I be sent to a breast center. It took time and effort, but finally, something went my way; I was referred to UCLA's Breast Center the very next day.

My doctors at UCLA were awesome and, yes, they actually looked at the infamous X-rays. I had my biopsy and it was determined that I had the early stages of breast cancer. The good news was that the cancer could be successfully treated. I was given two options for treatment. The first was to have surgery to remove the affected area (a lumpectomy) followed by another mammogram to be sure that the area had been cleaned out. I would then have one-hour radiation treatments, five days a week, for five consecutive weeks. There would be a seventy to eighty percent chance for success. My other option was to have a mastectomy with no follow-up treatment other than reconstructive surgery, if I wished.

I didn't spend much time crying or trying to figure out the cause; I just knew that I needed to resolve the problem as quickly as possible. I wasn't sick; I had always been a very healthy person—or so I thought. My body had been invaded, yet there were no symptoms, no pain, nothing to let me know that something was wrong. There was no lump and I had never heard of calcifications before.

And the questions, fears and doubts kept coming. So did the anger I felt toward the people and institutions that were supposed to be helping me. Cancer was on my mind 24/7.

But I knew almost from the start that I wanted to have a mastectomy and reconstructive surgery. Too much time had been wasted on dealing emotionally with something that had invaded my body and on getting the medical process started. I had to take control. I wanted this episode in my life to be over.

I had my mastectomy and reconstructive surgery on February 12, 1997. My road to that day and my recovery afterwards were rough, but I realized how much rougher they would have been were it not for the love and support of my family and friends. I felt sorry for patients I'd see alone in the doctor's office; what strength it must take to go it alone.

Everyone in my inner circle of "cancer confidants" was very supportive and protective of me. My husband came to appointments with me and we read and talked a lot about my cancer. My children were just as supportive, always giving me positive energy. I think my sister took it the hardest; but she sucked it up and was there for me, too. My very best friend was my sounding board and she helped in so many ways! I now know that the true test of friendship is being in the examining room with a friend while a plastic surgeon draws lines on her naked body. My best friend passed the test! And, of course, my mother, who has always considered herself a "prayerful person," busied herself doing her thing.

It's interesting how people are placed in your life for a specific reason, although you don't always realize their purpose at the time. No, I don't believe in coincidence and I'll tell you why. Five years prior to my diagnosis, a woman introduced herself to me at church when she realized that we lived in the same community. We had casual conversations when we ran into each other at the grocery store or at the mall, mostly talking about our children, church, and current events. We never visited each other's homes but considered ourselves friends.

I saw my friend one day at the cleaners and mentioned that I hadn't seen her at church in a while. She told me she had breast cancer and had had a mastectomy. Oh my God, I thought to myself, why is she sharing such personal information with me? Little did I know that what she was telling me was exactly what I would someday need to know for myself. When I got the results of my biopsy, she was the first person I called.

My friend was full of information and was very uplifting. She made me feel that I could conquer this and that's what I needed to hear. We talked frequently and her conversations helped me with my battle. When my doctor suggested that I join a support group, I remember asking my friend if she belonged to one and her response was, "Black folks don't go to support groups—we go to church!" I did attend one support group meeting for African-American women; I was the only one who showed up.

My friend, who had been so strong for me in my fight, lost her own battle with breast cancer in August, 1997. For me, it seemed that in her passing I had been channeled with the courage and love she had shown so many times. Along with her will, her support would carry me through my recovery and into the next chapter of my life as a "cancer survivor."

I use the term "cancer survivor" loosely because it sounds as if I was a passive participant in this battle for my life. I choose to believe that my heart, soul, spirit, faith, and positive attitude helped me win the fight against my cancer. I look at my experience as another bump in the road, not to minimize the experience but to acknowledge that life puts many obstacles in our paths.

Having cancer taught me to be a fighter, to be proactive, to be my own advocate. Now, I counsel others who are preparing for surgery. I've also come to realize recurrence is a possibility. When the doctor told me I was ninety-seven percent successfully treated, my thought was that there's no guarantee. But I'm not afraid. For the last six years, I've been blessed to cherish my life and the people in it, cancer-free.

BEVERLY PORTER

Kim

Kim, an OB/GYN nurse, just knew *she didn't have cancer. Yes, there was a small lump in her left breast, but because she had just had a baby, she and her doctor both believed the lump to be a clogged milk duct. Three years later, after the ordeal of surgery along with radiation and chemotherapy, her faith, family, and support group have helped her find the determination to continue her life journey.*

My name is Kim Collins. I have been a nurse for 13 years and am a breast cancer survivor. My story begins in the year 2000, when I was pregnant with my third daughter. In October, my husband found a lump in my breast about the size of a pea. During pregnancy, it's not uncommon for women to have lumpy breasts. However, on the next visit to my physician, I mentioned the lump. My physician checked it out and gave me a treatment regimen for a clogged milk duct.

From October 2000 to January 15, 2001 (when the baby was born), I followed my doctor's instructions, but the lump grew anyway. At delivery the lump was the size of a ping-pong ball. I tried to breastfeed, but absolutely nothing came out of that breast. I continued, as instructed by my physician, with the "clogged milk duct" treatments. During my eight-week postpartum visit (due to a C-section), we discovered that the lump had gotten bigger. At that point we both began to think this might be something other than a clogged milk duct.

Two weeks later, I had an ultrasound that was suspicious and was then scheduled for a mammogram. Because I was thirty-five, it was time for a baseline mammogram anyway. The mammography center was booked so I accepted the first available appointment. I knew there was a problem, but I was not in rush. The last thing I thought it could be was cancer.

After the mammogram, I waited for the radiologist to say, "all clear." Unfortunately, that's not what happened. Instead, the radiologist requested additional views and, by that evening, my doctor called me to come back in. The next day she told me her findings but never said the word cancer and I didn't think it. She said that I needed to see a surgeon, but the first available appointment was the last week of June.

At that point I became concerned. Driving home, I thought and thought. Having been an OB/GYN nurse since the early '90s, my experience and my human instinct told me, "This is serious, don't wait till June." When I got home I called the surgeon's office to reschedule. I was frustrated that they couldn't work me in the next day and I demanded an appointment within a week or less with whichever doctor in the group had an opening. I got it!

On June 5th, a couple of weeks after the mammogram, I had a breast biopsy. On my next doctor's visit a few days later, the doctor came in with two nurses and a box of tissues. I knew *exactly* what he was going to say. "It is cancer and it doesn't look good." My mom was with me and she completely lost it; the nurses ended up giving her the tissues and consolation. My initial response was pure shock, but I knew I couldn't lose it because decisions needed to be made. I called my husband on the cell phone so he could hear what the doctor had to say.

My physician recommended a left radical mastectomy ASAP. It was June and the lump was the size of a tennis ball. I was presented with the pathology report, which showed "Stage III, infiltrating duct carcinoma, suspicious for lymphatic invasion and positive for estrogen and progesterone receptors." I knew I was in serious trouble, so I scheduled surgery for the earliest date I could get. But my husband still wasn't comfortable with my decision, so (believe it or not) in a week's time we got four more opinions that all agreed with my surgeon's. Now my husband accepted the recommendation.

Then we went straight to our pastor and confided in her and asked for prayer. Later that night, it finally hit me. I just cried and couldn't stop. My husband and I cried and prayed together. How could this be? I knew God didn't give me this brand new baby only to say "good-bye." I knew I couldn't give up: I had to fight!

Now that there was no doubt, we had to tell our older girls. They cried, afraid that I would die. I simply told them to pray and ask God "to heal your mom and let her live." Then we called our siblings, who were very supportive.

My family members were there to support me on the day of my surgery. My baby brother came from northern Virginia, even though his wife was pregnant and having complications. Minutes before I was rolled into the O.R., my brother got an emergency call that the baby was coming. He had to leave. I recalled a statement commonly made by folks of the older generation: "When one goes out, one comes in." That sent butterflies into my stomach, but I went into surgery praying, "God please don't let me die." After a successful surgery, I heard God say, "All is well."

Two weeks post-op, I met with my oncologist who worked out a treatment plan: four treatments of Adriamycin™ and Cytoxin™, thirty-six chest wall radiation therapy sessions and then four Taxol™ treatments. My husband took me to all my treatments except the last round of chemo on February 1, 2002. I had the usual sickness with the treatments, but the worst experience was the hair loss. It devastated me. Most of my side-effects started four to six months after the last chemo: memory loss, fast growing cysts on my ovaries and uterus that led to a hysterectomy, and then Type 2 diabetes. We deal with the changes day-by-day and sometimes hour-by-hour, but we always put God first. My doctors say I am in remission, but I believe that I am almost healed.

One day at a fashion show I met a lady named Rita Ricks who introduced me to Sisters Network, a support group for breast cancer survivors, where I met other wonderful women, like Rose Thomas. Of course I joined the group. They didn't know me at first, yet they were so supportive with phone calls and cards. Sisters Network has truly been a blessing in my life. I can call them and talk about issues and not be considered crazy. Through all of this, I have definitely learned not to take life for granted. I thank God every day that I can see my girls and enjoy them. I thank God for a wonderful, more-than-supportive husband and a new group of friends within Sisters Network.

Chemotherapy, radiation, and seven surgeries later, I am still running for my life. *I shall not die but live!* Thanks for listening.

KIM COLLINS

Anna

For several months, the source of Anna's cancer was unknown. Eventually, she was diagnosed with a rare gynecological cancer at Stage Four. In addition to medial treatment Anna has taken a "four-pronged approach" to help heal herself: she changed her diet, exercises regularly, maintains a positive attitude and prays a lot.

Listen to your body and be persistent with your doctors.

During a three-month period I experienced painful swelling in my groin. My doctor initially treated me with antibiotics, but I later insisted that we attempt to find the cause of the swelling. The search for the cause of the swelling led me to several specialists and included countless tests and procedures. Finally, I met with an oncologist who noticed that the lymph nodes in my neck were also swollen. A biopsy revealed that I had cancer. I listened to the diagnosis, with my best friend by my side. The doctor told me that the cancer had also metastasized. There was also an additional concern—its primary source was unknown. I had a pad and was taking notes as the doctor spoke; trying to take it all in and bring an intellectual balance to an emotional situation. It seemed that I could not get home quickly enough. My family members were waiting for a call and when I spoke to my mother, it seemed as if I could hear her heart drop.

I was given a follow-up appointment to meet with the oncologists and a list of websites to learn more about the diagnosis. I had often heard the phrase, "first you cry . . ." but I never thought I would know the gravity of these words, firsthand. My family 'closed ranks' around me and let me know that 'we' were in this together. There was a frenzy of gathering information, getting a second opinion, taking more tests, and undergoing more procedures in an effort to determine the source of the cancer. I told my supervisor about my diagnosis because I anticipated major adjustments in my work schedule, but chose not to share this information with my colleagues. I needed time to absorb what was going on before I could feel comfortable telling others.

One month after receiving the initial diagnosis, I received the information we had all been searching for—fallopian tube cancer. Now that we knew what we were dealing with, a treatment plan was developed. But, I still had one person to tell—my daughter. It was probably one of the more difficult things I have ever done. My words were, "I have cancer and I need you to be on my team to help me fight it." We cried, and then we mobilized.

The oncologist and specialists proposed a treatment plan that included chemotherapy, surgery, and additional chemotherapy—with an evaluation at each phase. We talked openly about the affects of Carboplatin and Taxol®, about their experiences with women who had presented themselves as I did, and about my prognosis. These drugs were very strong, but aggressive measures were necessary, since the disease was at a Stage 4.

They never mentioned how I might be affected as a African-American compared to other women with gynecological cancers. I was told that everyone's biology is different, and they were not willing to make any predictions, so we would need to see how I responded to treatment. My team decided that in addition to medical treatment, mine would be a four-pronged approach to healing, which included a change in diet, regular exercise, maintaining a positive attitude, and prayer.

Except for my family members, I told only a few other people about my condition, but before long I was getting phone calls and e-mail messages from many other people who offered support, information, recommendations, and their prayers. I sought comfort from other resources. I joined an on-line group and began contacting the women that I knew who were cancer survivors. The online group did not last long. The conversations, for the most part, were not very encouraging. I canceled my subscription to the online group and decided to rely more on the women I knew who were cancer survivors. I needed to connect with people who were focused on living.

Prior to my first treatment, the doctor gave me a tour of the facility, introduced me to my nurse, and explained the procedure. Having this knowledge gave me a great sense of relief; I knew what to expect. I was placed on a 28-day cycle of chemotherapy that consisted of four and 1/2 hours of treatment, administered intravenously. My physical reaction to the first treatment was terrible. It seemed that I experienced every side effect possible to some extent, including nausea, a tingling sensation in my hands and feet, fatigue, constipation, loss of appetite, and loss of hair. These symptoms subsided after a few days and I then had a better sense of what I was dealing with.

It has always been helpful for me to write about my feelings. This was not different. I found comfort in journaling, meditation, and prayer. As for my appearance—the new diet and exercise regimen resulted in a slight weight loss and a more toned body. I now own more beautiful scarves, head wraps, and enjoy the convenience of wigs. Yet, each time I look in the mirror, I am confronted by my challenge.

I am adhering to the plan. My sister provided me with interesting recipes for my diet consisting mainly of fish, vegetables, and fruit; my daughter has joined a fitness class with me; my attitude remains positive, and my faith is still strong. Subsequent treatments have been manageable and the side effects have been minimal. I am responding well to treatment, the cancer levels are decreasing, my energy is good, and we are still on course.

When I was diagnosed with cancer, I thought a lot about death and the people who have gone before me. We don't get to choose our time to die, but we can choose to make the most of the time we have. So many clichés are rooted in truth. It has been five months since the diagnosis. I have just reached a point where I can talk about my condition, but I am still guarded. This experience has made me pay attention to life; it has helped me to learn more about making choices, establishing priorities, and finding the extraordinary in the ordinary, I am consciously, willingly learning about myself and my relation to others. I am enjoying today and looking forward to tomorrow.

ANNA LOWE

Melva

Melva was having the time of her life. She didn't have time for breast cancer, but the bump under her armpit kept growing and growing. Finally, pressure from family and co-workers forced her to get a mammogram. After the removal of three tumors, Melva now knows that you cannot ignore the signs of illness. Nor can you wish them away. She wants others to learn from her mistakes.

In 1988, I was diagnosed with breast cancer. Prior to the diagnosis, there were signs that I might have a problem, but I did not want to believe that it could be cancer. So I chose not to do anything.

The first sign was a small egg-like bump in my right armpit, which I spoke about with many of my friends and co-workers. They suggested that it was probably an infected hair follicle and advised me to change deodorants. So, I began to switch from Estée Lauder™, Sure™, Mum™, Arid™, Secret™, and Right Guard™, but the lump grew and grew. One day I asked a co-worker to remove the hair from the bump. She started crying and sobbing and finally she yelled, "You have to be seen today by MD Anderson, now!" Well, I did not want to hear her because I had a great job, I was running in the fast lane, and I was having loads of fun. I did not have time for breast cancer.

Eventually, under pressure from many people, I went to MD Anderson, a cancer center affiliated with the University of Texas in Houston, Texas. Doctors there advised me to have surgery, but I delayed it because I did not want to worry my son, who was graduating from high school. On June 6, 1980, I had a mastectomy. Three tumors were removed.

Although my future looked gloomy, I now thank God for allowing me to have breast cancer. I now know what faith really is and how God can heal, no matter what the prognosis is. New-found relationships with my family have developed and that feels good. My husband spoils me to no end.

Recovery was not easy. I had chemotherapy, which resulted in hair loss, mouth sores, nausea, and vomiting. However, I believe that I came out smelling like a rose. I did great and continue to do so. I now understand that ignoring the signs of cancer will not make it go away. I am now more proactive when it comes to my health.

I was approached by a social worker and asked if I would participate in a clinical trial at MD Anderson. There was no hesitation from me in saying yes because I wanted the benefits that accompany the project—social support, nutrition training, cancer updates, access to a regular team of physicians and nurses, and involvement in ongoing research. All of my health needs are met, including Pap tests, colonoscopies, breast cancer follow-ups, and medicine. The health care team is just a phone call away and they always return my calls.

I really want to be a tool of support and help to others. If my research team learns anything that will aid in prevention or ultimate cure, then I will feel good knowing that my involvement aided in the process. This is a great hospital. I like my team and I enjoy the visits.

I have also become a member of a support group called the "Victorious Ones" and I am participating in the "Celebrating Life Foundation," both in Dallas. I also continue to work.

There is life after breast cancer. It is okay to be afraid, but not okay to ignore the signs. Because I ignored the signs of the illness, I caused financial hardship for my family and enabled the cancer to spread. Overall, I have learned a lot from this process.

MELVA STEPHENS

CHAPTER THREE

Timing

"EVERY [PERSON] IS BORN INTO THE WORLD TO DO
SOMETHING UNIQUE AND SOMETHING DISTINCTIVE, AND
IF SHE DOES NOT DO IT, IT WILL NEVER BE DONE."

—Benjamin Rays, *I Knew Carter G. Woodson*

Ceyeka

Cekeya, a nineteen-year-old college student, was a thousand miles from home when she learned she had Hodgkin's Lymphoma. Unable to get support from an incarcerated father or a mother she didn't get along with, she found it elsewhere, especially in her church, where she had learned that "we can overcome by the words of our testimony." In the diary she kept throughout the treatment process, she actualized that teaching.

I am a nineteen-year-old Hodgkin's Lymphoma survivor. I am also a student who is determined to complete my college education. I was raised in a single-parent home; my father was incarcerated and I have a strained relationship with my mother. Yes, though I'm young, I have fallen and I have risen. I have encountered many of life's obstacles, but I will always use the lessons I learn as tools for success in my future.

I entered a world full of new challenges and high expectations when I went away to college. Although my first year at Xavier University in New Orleans was difficult, it turned out to be a great adventure. I had to overcome the fear of being a freshman. Sometimes I felt like I really wasn't there. Although I was an out-of-state student who really didn't know anyone, I gave it my best effort.

At school I became involved with clubs and organizations such as the Pre-Law Club, Gospel Choir, and the Pre-Alumni Counsel. I found a job and a new church home. I took charge of my life and tried to make decisions that would lead to positive results.

By the middle of the summer of 2002, I began to feel fatigued and to have headaches. A lump appeared on my neck. I immediately went to the doctor and, on August 28, 2002, I was diagnosed with Hodgkin's Lymphoma. Under doctor's orders, I did not work or attend school for the Fall 2002 and Spring 2003 semesters. The doctor also advised me to return to California for chemotherapy treatments.

The treatments were given every other week for five hours at a time. During this period, I became much closer to God and, with determination, support from family, friends, and my brothers and sisters in Christ, I made it through. I continued to attend church and joined a support group to meet with other cancer patients. Throughout my ordeal, I continued to study for school.

As of March 3, 2003, I successfully completed chemotherapy. Now, as a first-generation college student, I am determined to do whatever it takes to finish my education.

I am thankful for my experience with cancer because it has taught me how to appreciate people for who they are. It has also taught me not to take things such as life and health for granted. I am committed to making a change in the lives of those I come in contact with, by listening and being supportive in any way possible. I will also inform anyone who will listen about my story and how regular check-ups are important.

I have overcome so many personal and family obstacles in my life. I feel proud to say I never let those tribulations make me give up. My experiences as a child growing up alone, with no support in the home, have actually given me the motivation to achieve great things.

Growing up in church, I was taught we can overcome by the words of our testimony. By developing my own personal relationship with God and going through the treatment process, I have realized that the teaching is true. At this point in time, I am back at Xavier in New Orleans. Praise the Lord. *Keep God first!*

CEKEYA GILBERT

Theresa

Theresa's three-year old daughter lay on the cold floor snoring, as she had been doing a lot. Theresa's doctor told her that it was nothing but an ear infection. But after the child continued to experience rapid weight loss, Theresa, who had trusted her doctor, knew that something was seriously wrong. But what?

My daughter was only three and a half years old when she was diagnosed with leukemia. I did not know right away that she had cancer. In the beginning, I noticed that she began to snore and was losing weight. I figured that she was just sick. I took her to the doctor a few days later and was told that she had an ear infection. We were given antibiotics and sent home. After seven to ten days, she appeared to be alright—but she was still losing weight. I could see her bones through her skin.

One day, she began bleeding heavily after a cut. The bleeding eventually stopped, but I was still concerned. A few days later, she looked sick again and would not eat. She was losing weight and sleeping even more. Again I took her to the doctor and told him everything that was going on. He still did not order X-rays or blood tests because he thought she had a throat infection. Now, this is a child that had never been sick, not at birth or during her first few years. Why was she sick now? I, not knowing, but being a concerned parent, accepted this information. This was a certified doctor who should have been able to diagnose an illness.

During this time, my family and I decided to move and my daughter and I stayed for a week at a relative's house. While we were there, my child ate very little. Then she did the most bizarre thing: She just laid on the cold floor and slept, snoring very loudly. I explained to my family what was going on and they suggested that I take her to their hospital, which I did. The doctor who examined her said that she may have the mumps. Her lymph nodes appeared to stand out of her body. I told them about my ordeal with this sick child so the physician ordered a blood test. When the doctors saw that her blood was like water, they immediately ordered X-rays. The X-rays showed large masses of cancer covering her lungs. She was finally admitted to the hospital and assigned a specialist. I was on an emotional rollercoaster. The specialist who diagnosed my daughter told me things I could not understand. My emotions were mixed. "Is she dying? Why us? *Why!*"

My daughter was immediately sent to one of the best hospitals for cancer research, where she was put on antibiotics. The specialist explained that she needed intensive chemotherapy because she had been diagnosed so late. He said he was surprised that she was still alive. I cried for hours that night. The next couple of years were crucial. All the questions about the family history of cancer and other illnesses were taken into consideration as she was being treated.

Six years of our lives were put on hold. I went through fifty different emotions a day and for the first few years, I blamed myself. I kept saying, "If only I had known the warning signs, I would have done things differently. Maybe if she had better insurance and was not receiving Medicaid she would have gotten better care at first."

Cancer almost took the life of my child. I realized that I had to become educated, especially because of other problems that were associated with this illness. My daughter had to go through many blood transfusions, three surgeries, chemotherapy, radiation, yeast growing in her blood, and many, many other issues. I did not think that I could go on, but I did.

My daughter is now a budding thirteen-year-old. She gets her heart checked once a year because of the side effects from one of the types of chemotherapy she had. She also goes once a year for a physical to make sure everything is okay. She is developmentally delayed about three years from the radiation treatments to her brain and skull area. Other than that, she is a happy child with the same issues as other thirteen-year-olds. When you look at her, you would not know that she had ever had cancer.

When I thought my ordeal with cancer was finally over, my father was diagnosed with colon cancer. Because of the experience with my daughter, I advised him on where to get help. He did not follow my advice because he was secure in his choice of care, but eventually, my father died. Before he passed away, I saw him lying in a bed. I also saw my daughter lying in that same bed that he lay in. He looked like a little boy. He eventually had a silent stroke that took away his speech, sight, and everything that I associated with him. He would not respond to anyone and would not move. When I whispered to him that it was Theresa and I loved him, he acknowledged that I was there. I had hope. He died the next day, July 3, 2003. Some say that he was hanging in there for me but I know that God knew what he was doing. He is in a better place now.

It is imperative that people of color get checked for cancer. Not knowing can have devastating consequences.

THERESA BELL-LIAS

Pamela

Five-year old Li'l Charlie was special. He gave his parents and everyone around him joy and happiness. When he was two, his doctor found a tumor the size of a baseball near his kidney.

No, not again! If *Reader's Digest* magazine was a hard-backed book, my slamming it closed could have been mistaken for an earthquake. Here I go again, I thought. I just can't read another article about a small child suffering with and ultimately dying of cancer or some other disease—not again.

Memories of the first time I read a story in *Reader's Digest* about a dying child, before my own son's illness and death, came back to haunt me. I had cried and cried as I read about the beautiful young daughter of loving parents who was dying of cystic fibrosis. After every page I was compelled to pause, cry, and think about how hard it must have been for her parents to see their daughter suffer with such a horrible illness, one that ultimately took her young life. I thought of my own son who had just turned five years old and about how much I loved him. My heart went out to these people whom I only knew through a magazine story. Little did I know that the article could have been written by me a few months later.

"Is there a history of cancer in your family?" That was the question that changed the course of my life forever. "No, why?" I asked my estranged husband the same question. It was his weekend to be entertained by our smart, loving, kind-hearted, and over-protective son who had been named after his father. "They think Li'l Charlie has a cancerous tumor on his kidney."

All I could think about was the article in *Reader's Digest*. Now it was my turn. I thought I should never have read that stupid article. I felt like I had been jinxed.

At the hospital, I was told that the doctor wanted to speak with me before I saw Li'l Charlie. There it was, right on the X-ray, blocking the view between Li'l Charlie's ribs. "It's about the size of a baseball," I remember Doctor Whatever-His-Name-Was telling me. "We'll have to admit him immediately to our facility in Hollywood, where he can be under a pediatric oncologist's care. He'll be okay. We can get it and he'll be good as new!" Why? Why, God, why? Why did I have to read that stupid article in *Reader's Digest?* I had to blame someone or something—nothing was off-limits, not even God or a stupid article.

Through my beautiful son's illness and his walk with death, a walk I prayed I could take for him and if not, at least with him, I learned how strong young, sick children can be. Although he seemed to take everything in stride, nothing, absolutely nothing, could ease the agony, torment, guilt, and hatred that festered inside of me. For three months, I watched my only child's life being slowly taken away. Through this time, he was constantly uplifting me, telling me not to worry, soon he would be okay. I realize now that he accepted his impending death long before I did.

"Mom, tell them to stop sticking me with those needles. I don't want them anymore," I remember him saying about a week before he died. I knew then that he was ready to let go of life on Earth and begin his trip to Heaven.

There were no beds for parents in the hospital rooms, so I rested and slept upright in a chair beside Li'l Charlie's bed. I would sit in that chair for hours, just watching him awaken and sleep. Li'l Charlie looked so peaceful when he slept, like God was smiling upon him. Even though he lost weight, he never looked like a dying child, at least not in my eyes.

The night before Li'l Charlie died I was awakened by a strong voice demanding, "Mom, go home and get some sleep. I'll be okay." I didn't want to go home, but Li'l Charlie was insistent and appeared to get upset when I would not leave. I told him okay, but I would be back in few hours. I did come back, after I received a telephone call stating that Li'l Charlie was slipping away and that I should hurry. As I ran to his room and put my hand on the door to enter, I was suddenly stopped by one of the nurses. "Wait," she said, "I have to tell you something. He's already gone." I fell to my knees gasping for air. The only thing I vividly remember is calling on God to help me through this and to fulfill His promise that He would never leave me or forsake me.

Three months after burying Li'l Charlie, I discovered that I was pregnant. I was devastated. Instead of celebrating the blessing, my first thoughts were that I would not let another child suffer again. The only way to be certain of this was not to have another child. Without hesitation, I decided to have an abortion.

Then it happened. The miracle of the Holy Ghost spoke to my heart and spirit, saying, "How could you be so devastated over the death of one child and yet contemplate killing another?" I thought about how I had called on Him to help me through the pain of losing Li'l Charlie. It suddenly became clear to me that when I called on God, I did not ask Him to let me direct my path but asked that He direct my path. I realized that I put Him in charge of my life and my pregnancy was part of his answer.

Today, Latiesha is a God-loving, healthy, talented, and compassionate young woman. She did not take the place of Li'l Charlie—that is not her purpose here.

Li'l Charlie's life had a purpose, and his memory and purpose live on through These Three Words, an organization that assists needy families of terminally-ill children. I co-founded it with another mother of a deceased child.

Now, when I think about the article *in Reader's Digest,* I no longer wonder where the parents of that particular dying child found the strength to live on. I now know where—the same place I did, through God.

PAMELA AUSTIN-LOCKHART

Adrienne

Adrienne's ovarian cancer was discovered during a pregnancy in which she miscarried. Then during a second pregnancy, her oncologist told her she would need chemotherapy that could threaten the fetus. She was shattered. But for Adrienne, the miracle was just beginning.

My name is Adrienne Moore. I am a 32-year-old African-American female and I am overjoyed to share my story with you.

I have a truly miraculous survivor story, although I do understand that *all* stories of survival are miracles. We certainly should all live each day with that in mind.

In February of 2003, I discovered that I was pregnant. My fiancé and I had been planning a September wedding and were taken aback by the news. We were not actually disappointed about the pregnancy, but it just wasn't in our plans. We had used the same method of birth control since we began dating and never once had a pregnancy scare. Still, we knew we had to change the wedding date and have a less elaborate wedding than we had originally planned.

Over the next month, I psyched myself up about being pregnant and was looking forward to having a child. At 11 weeks, I started to spot. I had not had my first OB appointment yet. Frightened, my fiancé and I spent six hours in the emergency room. At first the doctors believed that I had an ectopic pregnancy. They were curious about the empty yolk sac in my uterus and the large mass that seemed to be in my fallopian tube. Twins maybe, but not salvageable. I was told I needed surgery.

I couldn't believe it. God, I was prepared for a simple miscarriage but what was this? When I called the surgeon (God's life-saving instrument), he told me that there was some type of mass on my left ovary. He was scheduling me for a D&C that week. However, there was no baby. I was crushed. Was there something wrong with my body that I could produce a yolk sac with no baby?

Before the surgery, the doctor assured me of a simple in-and-out procedure to remove what he said was a non-malignant mass from my ovary. He mentioned the word "cancer" a few times but was explicit in saying that because I was so young, he was not too concerned about cancer. On the day of the surgery he confirmed that we were dealing with a benign entity, but that now he *did* have to remove my left ovary and part of the fallopian tube.

Two weeks later I learned that under microscopic examination a few indifferential cells had been discovered. My doctor called my home at 8:30 on a Tuesday evening to break the news to me that we were indeed dealing with a cancerous tumor. Without actually staging, the pathologist felt we were dealing with Stage II ovarian cancer. What the . . . ?

I immediately looked for any information I could find on it. It must be simple, I thought, treatable. One hardly ever hears of ovarian cancer and I soon found out why. They call ovarian "the whisper" because it has quiet symptoms or none at all. The majority of cases are diagnosed in the advanced stages when it has spread to other reproductive organs, throughout the pelvic floor and into the bowels. The prognosis knocked my legs out from under me. I was only thirty-two years old. Is this how I was going to die? My God, my God. I must have prayed and lain on my face for hours over the next few days. Save me, Father, I prayed, save Your child.

A second surgery was scheduled to determine whether the cancer had spread. Initially the oncologist felt that if it had not, chemotherapy would not be necessary. My oncologist was optimistic because we had caught the cancer early enough for it to be treated with the standard protocol.

My Heavenly Father, however, had other plans for His daughter. One day as I was praying, I truly felt that the last tear of worry had fallen from my face. I got up with a peaceful, calm feeling, believing that I was going to be fine. The cancer had not spread and there would be no chemotherapy. God told me that. It came to me so clearly.

I realized that I had to become pregnant so that an ultrasound would be done. This is the only way this type of cancer can be diagnosed early. God had been working this out all along. Now, I was focused. I realized I had been looking at my circumstances but not at the God of my circumstances. I was praying for Him to change them when, in actuality, He had ordered and resolved them in one. "Holy, Holy." That's a testimony.

On May 16, 2003, my oncologist told my family that I was clear of cancer. But the story doesn't end there. I still needed chemotherapy. I was to start treatment on June 18, one month after my surgery. I was quite disappointed. I wanted it to be over. And, besides, that's not what God had told me. He had said, "No more surgery, no chemo," and He is always true to His word. On June 13, something came over me and I decided to take a pregnancy test. It was positive! But how could that be? On June 15, the same OB/GYN who performed my first surgery did an ultrasound and confirmed my pregnancy. He immediately spoke with the oncologist who agreed they would not terminate my pregnancy so that I could have chemotherapy. They would, however, remove my right ovary at the time of delivery to reduce my chance of recurrence. That's how that could be. God was not through with me yet.

I am now twelve weeks pregnant and we are getting married on August 29th. Although I have left out many details, I am thankful to all my friends and family members who prayed for me and gave me support through this time, especially my wonderful fiancé. But nothing can match the joy I feel knowing that God is God of all things, all the time and knowing most of all that He loves me. There is no better feeling.

ADRIENNE MOORE

CHAPTER FOUR

Choices

I LEARNED THAT I PERHAPS WAS LEADING A LIFE
THAT WAS TOO STRESSFUL, AND THAT I NEEDED TO
STOP AND SMELL THE ROSES A LITTLE BIT.

—Ben Carson, on *Good Morning America*

Kat

Kat was already into taking care of her health and alternative therapies, so when she was diagnosed with breast cancer, she decided to take her treatment into her own hands. Her courage and tenacity deepened her spiritual growth and her will to succeed.

I was diagnosed with breast cancer in September of 2000. Shock does not even come close to the feeling I had after being told that my lump was a malignant mixed tumor. I was someone who regularly fasted, ate well, and took supplements. I considered myself generally, healthy. Several months before the diagnosis, I had become anemic and hypoglycemic, which led me to get a physical. Instead of freaking out, I went into warrior mode. Because I had an affinity for alternative medicine, I read as much about alternatives as I did conventional treatment. I had a lumpectomy in October and the doctors suggested that I have radiation and chemotherapy. I am a singer by profession. When the doctors told me that medications like Tamoxifen™, used in chemotherapy, could damage my voice, I refused to do the follow-up treatments. By then I had read so much about alternatives that I thought I could find a miracle after surgery. I went to several alternative clinics, where I received intravenous vitamin therapy, bio-ray, saunas, mistletoe extract shots, liver shots (for the anemia), and light therapy. By March, I had spent almost $10,000 and still didn't feel I was completely safe.

At the New York Health Expo, I met an Asian woman I will call Ann, who sold me an infrared heating device called the Onnetsuki. Ann had written a book on overcoming cancer, in which she talked about a clinic in Japan that was supposedly curing various types of cancer using the device. When Ann worked on me, the area where the cancer had been found became extremely hot. She told me it was hot because the cancer was still there. After treatment for three weeks, the area no longer got hot. I bought the Onnetsuki for $800. I am not sure to this day how it works.

Feeling as though I had found a home at Ann's treatment center, I stopped taking vitamin drips and other treatments because she convinced me that I no longer needed them. She said I didn't need to get a mammogram because the Onnetsuki was also a detection device. That summer I went to Japan with her for a healing retreat at "The Shinkiko Healing Center," which based healing on energy. The device they used was called the "Hi

Genki." It supposedly deals with stagnant energy so that good energy can flow and revitalize the body. It cost over $2,000 but hey, I thought, that's a worthwhile investment to keep myself alive.

For the next six months I used the Onnetsuki and Hi Genki daily to prevent recurrence. But unfortunately, my lump came back in the same area. I will never forget turning over in bed and feeling the mass again; it felt harder than before and maybe even bigger. Of course when I went to Ann, she told me she could treat it in 3 weeks costing me almost $1,000. I was even more devastated the second time because my fear now was that I had ignored the doctors and I might have to do harsher treatment like complete breast removal and stronger chemo. I did more research and found another alternative therapy called "escharotics."

A practitioner named Dan had been using escharotics (bloodroot paste) on skin and breast cancers for ten years with a high level of success. At this point, I felt I had nothing to lose. If it didn't work, I would acquiesce and do whatever the doctors told me to do.

On my first day of using the escharotics, I felt a burning sensation and after twenty-four hours, the skin of the treated area turned black. By the second day, I felt a yanking and pulling as though the treatment were drawing something up. By the fourth day, I was in so much pain it was hard to get out of bed. The skin had opened up and a lot of "matter" was coming out.

All I could think was that if I went to my conventional doctors now they would check me into a psych ward. For some reason, though I was in intense pain, I had an internal feeling that the area was really being disinfected of the bad cells. I could feel the pain all the way down to my lungs. By the eighth day, I was told to stop using the bloodroot, to switch to Vaseline, and to allow the area to heal because my lump was gone. My breast was sore and swollen, but to feel confident. I allowed it to heal for a few months so that I could get a mammogram.

I have to say that before the mammogram, the area felt lump-free and believe me, I have learned to dig for lumps. When the radiologists told me my mammogram was perfectly clear, I jumped for joy! Not only was the cancer undetected, I was also clear of anemia and hypoglycemia. For the first time in years, I actually felt healthy.

It has been two years since my bloodroot treatment. My breast still feels lump-free, but regardless, I am going for my mammogram later on this month. Some may think I am crazy, but if another lump were found in another area, I would probably do the escharotics again. There is a voice in my head, however, that doubts I will ever have to deal with breast cancer again.

Having cancer gave me the opportunity to really question the spiritual and physical realms of our lives. What I came up with is this: there are a lot of things we just don't understand and maybe never will. I think I learned to accept that, but not to accept giving up.

KATREESE BARNES

Anesha

Anesha discovered she had breast cancer a month before her thirtieth birthday. One doctor recommended a complete mastectomy, followed by chemotherapy. She didn't want either treatment. She selected a regimen of spiritual therapy, combined with vitamin and fasting therapies. Now she believes she's changed her life for the better.

When I received the call from the doctor stating that the tumor in my breast was cancerous, I thought, "This can't be happening to me . . . I'm too young . . . this disease doesn't even run in my family." My mother, sister, niece, and I held one another's hands and began to pray.

The tumor was small. Because it was discovered at an early stage, I thought I could simply have it cut out and then the whole ordeal would be over. My doctors, however, thought otherwise. The first doctor recommended that I undergo a complete mastectomy. Uneasy with this course of action, I got a second opinion. The second doctor felt that in my case, it was not necessary to remove the entire breast. She opted for having the tumor removed with chemotherapy to follow. Not wanting to have my breast removed or to undergo chemotherapy, I decided to go the alternative medicine route.

The day after I received the first doctor's recommendation, I woke up feeling helpless, alone, and scared. I felt that my life was over. I tried holding back the tears because I didn't want my family to see the mental state I was really in. I didn't want them to worry about me.

I turned on the television, began flipping channels and came across a program that appeared to be a debate of some sort between two men, one on either side of a table. Normally I would not have given a show like that a second look, but I felt compelled to continue watching this one. One of the gentlemen was Robert Barefoot. He was talking about a supplement by the name of coral calcium that, he said, was known to reverse diseases such as cancer. Mr. Barefoot said that the body can repair and heal itself when given the right elements to do so. I knew instantly it was no one but God who had caused me to turn on the television when I did and who guided me to that particular station. That morning was the last time I ever felt defeated by cancer.

My body was deficient in something and I needed to know

what that was in order to equip it to fight back. I began taking coral calcium and also sought the help of Elliott Sterling, a holistic doctor in Houston. Elliott believes that all diseases stem from negative emotions. Because the tumor was in my left breast, Elliott said, my cancer resulted from emotional wounds caused by a woman. I had no idea what he was talking about. I have always had close relationships with my mother and sister. Outside my family, I was well-liked and had no enemies. I could not recall ever having been emotionally wounded by a female. A man or men, yes, but not a woman. Despite being unable to recall a person or event, I asked God to cleanse my heart and to help me forgive the individual or individuals who may have done me harm.

After getting myself right psychologically, I began to work on the physiological. I changed my diet and became a vegetarian for a four-month period. Eventually, I went on a six-week liquid fast, the Breuss fast. This detox and purification program required that I drink a particular vegetable juice and certain teas. Nothing but the grace of God sustained me during that time and He has continued to sustain me. My weight dropped to 88 pounds during the detox and purification. After I successfully completed the fast, I resumed eating and incorporated lean meats (turkey, fish, and chicken) back into my diet.

In approximately three weeks it will be a year since I received the call that changed my life—for the better. I have a new take on life. I eat a healthier diet and forgave those who may have caused me pain. Maybe this happened so that I could help others by sharing my testimony. We don't always go through trials for ourselves. Sometimes we go through trials for others.

No weapon formed against me *shall prosper* (Isaiah 54:17).

ANESHA EVANS

Thomasina

Thomasina believed she was in peak health until she got the results of her colonoscopy. These are the lessons she learned from her cancer experience that she wants to share with you:

- Never take your health for granted.
- Be sensitive to changes in your body.
- Educate yourself about how your body works and how to keep it healthy.
- Take charge of your health by having regular medical check-ups and tests.
- Encourage others to follow this formula, to prevent disease or catch it early.

I am 59-years-old—and was advised by my primary physician for several years to have a colon cancer test. It was considered part of the standard group of preventive tests that my healthcare provider encouraged. I had no family history of colon cancer so I did not feel any urgency.

After I retired in early 2002, I decided to have a test done. This test is called a flex sigmoid and is performed by inserting a lighted tube through the rectum into the lower colon. The patient is awake and, along with the doctor, is able to see the colon on a screen similar to a television. For most people it is only mildly uncomfortable.

I was shocked when my doctor pointed out what he said was cancerous growth on the wall of my colon. It looked innocent enough and I questioned my doctor's diagnosis. The attending physician also thought the growth had the appearance of cancer, although further testing was needed. A colonoscopy followed a couple of days later and the diagnosis was confirmed.

I was lucky. Although I was diagnosed with Stage III colon cancer, only two lymph nodes were involved, one visibly detectable by the surgeon and another detected by biopsy. In addition, the cancer had not spread to any of my organs. My treatment consisted of six months of chemotherapy. I have been tested twice since completing chemo and appear to be cancer-free at this time.

My doctor informed me that my cancer was a "slow grower" and had probably been "in process" for several years before detection. Until the cancer diagnosis I never had any real health issues. In fact, my doctor always told me how healthy I was each year when I went in for my annual physical.

Were there any indications that I should have been aware of? Yes, but they were subtle. I lost ten pounds in one year, but I had been trying to lose a few pounds. Finally a real red flag: I noticed blood on my tissue after bowel movements a week before my scheduled test. Alarmed, I called my doctor, who questioned me regarding additional symptoms and concluded that I might have a hemorrhoid that would be detected during testing.

We are all guilty of making our health a low priority until we receive a jolt that changes our perspective. My message is: make no assumptions regarding your health! Please take the time to be tested! Do everything that you can to assure your continued quality of life. Be proactive, ask questions, and be informed. Be sensitive to your body. Know when anything changes or just does not feel quite right. You may save your life.

THOMASINA ELLIS

Sheila

Sheila was determined to bring joy and strength back into her life after the devastating news of her malignant tumor. She overcame her hair loss and psychological turmoil to find beauty in her family, friends, and surroundings once again.

At age 36 I was diagnosed with cancer. Everything I had ever read and heard prior to my diagnosis had convinced me that I didn't need to worry about breast cancer, at least until I reached the age of 40. Because I was not concerned about breast cancer, I was not doing self-exams on a regular basis. But one day in the shower, a little voice said to me, "Shelia, check yourself, " and there it was. I knew in my heart what it was but I waited a couple of months before I scheduled my doctor's appointment. I wanted to let my family enjoy their Christmas.

My family doctor did a clinical exam as part of my regular yearly physical; I did not mention the lump in my breast. And, guess what, she missed the lump—I had to show her where it was. She told me that she was almost certain that it was nothing, that I was too young to have breast cancer. But I insisted that it be checked and removed.

When I went to the surgeon for the results of my biopsy, he walked in with tears in his eyes and I knew that this was not going to be an ordinary day for me. I screamed out and began to cry. Then I dropped to my knees in prayer as the nurse and the doctor left the room. When I got up off my knees, it seemed as if a lot of time had passed and I knew that from that point on that everything was in God's hands.

I learned something new when I heard the three words, "You have cancer. " I learned how strong my faith in God was. All my life I had been looking for my higher purpose, wanting to do things that would make a difference. Never did I dream that hearing those three words—"You have cancer"—could help me make a difference. Oddly enough, I can say now that I am a better person having heard those three words.

I don't remember much about the first week after being diagnosed except constantly praying the 23rd Psalm. Fear was trying to consume me. I cleaned and rearranged everything in my house. At times, as I moved from room to room, waves of fear came over me . . . so I prayed. I prayed for strength and I prayed for more time to see my two children grow into adulthood and be able to take care of themselves. I prayed for mercy.

God sent me several angels during my journey. The first one was my boss. She was in Atlanta at a conference when she learned that I was scheduled to have surgery. She called me and said, "Sheila, this is your life and I can't tell you what to do, but please seek a second opinion. I have someone you need to meet." I took her advice and called Dr. Terry Sarantou. Although he was very busy he saw me that same day. When he walked into the examining room, I felt a burden being lifted off my shoulders. He was my second angel and I knew that everything was going to be alright—he was a vessel being used by God.

I started aggressive treatment immediately. My doctor warned me that I would lose my hair and I did. I never thought I was a vain person and I was not the type to run to the beauty parlor on a regular basis—a ponytail was fine with me most of the time. But when my hair started falling out, I was devastated. So I shaved my head to save myself the pain of constantly pulling it out or finding it in my shower. I basically stopped looking in the mirror if I could help it, because when I did I didn't see Shelia—I saw a person with no eyelashes, no eyebrows and a bald head.

I bought a wig that I wore to work to make everyone else comfortable, but my co-workers knew that I would pull it off the moment it started to bother me. That wig spent so much time on the floorboard of my car that it could never be used by anyone else. I saw many shocked faces as I drove up Interstate 40 with my windows down and my shiny bald head. I was able to work throughout treatment and despite the bald head, my life was as normal as was possible given the circumstances.

After I finished chemotherapy, I tried to establish a support group with an already existing organization, but was told that I needed to wait until I had healed emotionally before they would grant my request. I was upset at first because I really needed a support group, but they were right. At the one-year mark I had an abnormal mammogram—and a total emotional breakdown.

On the outside I looked fine, but inside I was in turmoil. All I could think was "Not again, I can't do this again." This is when I met another one of my angels, Jocinta Williams. Ironically, we were both being prepared for surgery and were seated together in the waiting room. I was a mess but she smiled and spoke to me as I slid into a corner chair of the pre-op area. I never imagined that that chance meeting would form the basis of our friendship today.

After the second mammogram scare, a co-worker thought that I could inspire other Black women to speak openly about the disease. She wrote an article in the local paper about my journey. Because of this article I was contacted by a number of very special people, including Jocinta Williams and the local Susan G. Komen Foundation.

Now my life is fuller than it has ever been. Because of my journey, I have met many special people and have learned to love more openly and completely. I have learned to separate the pebbles from the sand and appreciate the tiniest things that come along with each day.

Three years ago, I would not have imagined myself in the place that I am now. Now I'm a mother who has stopped taking herself too seriously and who dances and sings with her children. I'm also a person who realizes the beauty of the clouds and the rain and a person who enjoys the wonderful closeness of friends and family. Now I know the joy of laughter and have strength in my life again.

SHEILA MOORE

CHAPTER FIVE

What's Race Got To Do With It?

SURGERY WENT WELL, VERY WELL. I'M WELL INTO
THE RECOVERY PERIOD. AND IT JUST REMINDS ALL OF
US THAT PROSTATE CANCER IS A SERIOUS MATTER FOR
MEN, AND ESPECIALLY FOR BLACK MEN.

—Colin Powell, *Nightline*

I HOPE THAT WE WILL DEMAND THAT BLACK WOMEN
GET CHECKED ON A YEARLY BASIS—THE MINIMUM
THAT WE MUST DO TO TAKE CARE OF OURSELVES, AND
SOME OF US SHOULD GO TWICE A YEAR. THERE IS A
GREAT TENDENCY TO BE CARETAKERS AMONG BLACK
AMERICAN WOMEN. WHILE THAT IS TO BE ADMIRED,
NEGLECTING OURSELVES IS JUST NOT ACCEPTABLE.

—Diahann Carroll, *USA Today*

D. T. Negrin

D. T. Negrin looked directly at her life and her disease and didn't blink. Because she comes from a family of cancer survivors, she knew what to expect. She also understood that as an African-American woman she had special resources for fighting cancer. Certainly she did! She has been cancer free for thirteen years.

I've often thought of myself as different—not your typical cancer patient. I approached my treatment and recovery with an attitude of independence and self-reliance. I knew exactly how I would react the moment I heard the diagnosis: what I would feel and what I would do. My reaction to the doctor's words was as predictable as my daily morning routine. After all, I had witnessed the cancer ritual many, many times in my life.

My mother and her two sisters had been diagnosed with breast cancer. It would be my turn next. This would be just one of those things. I would simply follow the doctor's instructions, as long as I thought they were what was best for me, and move on with my life. Being an African-American woman, was this really the worst thing that could happen to me? This cancer thing was really no big deal. My attitude was critical to my healing, as critical as any therapy, any doctor's advice. This was no mask. This was how I felt and continue to feel. I didn't want anyone feeling sorry for me. I couldn't use their pity and it would only prolong the healing process.

My doctors, nurses, and medical technicians kept telling me that I was in denial because I was taking it all in stride. But that's just how I am. Even at home in my solitude, as I looked at the four walls, listened to music, watched TV, cooked, and cleaned, I knew that I would be alright.

I think healing requires the nurturing of the spirit, the mind, and the body. Perhaps there is a gene that causes the cancer to be more aggressive in African-American women. I don't know. But I don't believe that that's particularly important. Too often for African-American women, the mind and spirit are not integral parts of their treatment plans. Healing is a holistic process.

Of course, my doctor didn't talk to me about a plan of treatment that was specifically for African-American women. But isn't that just like everything else in this society? What I found out, I discovered on my own.

During treatment, my hair fell out. We African American people—men, women and children—have such a complex relationship with our hair. We fry it, dye it, twist it, perm it, weave some on, take some off—anything to make it different from what it is. Now, my hair was lying on the floor. I thought about it every time I put that wig on. Lucky me. I didn't have to comb it anymore. I grew to love my wig even when it was just a little twisted on my head.

I've lived my life not really worrying about what other people think. I told my friends about my cancer. They love me. I didn't care what other people thought about it or what they think now. As an African American person, I've had a lot of practice being tough, especially when I didn't feel like it.

D.T. NEGRIN

Ruth

Dr. Ruth King is an educational psychologist, a founding member of a writer's group, and a practitioner of the Yang style of Tai Chi Chuan. She characterizes herself as "a feisty senior citizen," and this attitude, along with her healthy lifestyle, has helped her conquer the challenges she faced after being diagnosed with breast cancer.

I was 71 years of age when a routine mammogram detected a small lump in my breast. I actually received a letter in the mail saying that there was some irregularity and I thought they meant with the test, not me. I was highly annoyed, so it took a while for me to go back in and have another test. After the second test was completed, I received a telephone call (not a letter this time) telling me that a lump had been discovered in my right breast and that I had to come for a sonogram.

I didn't know anything about breast cancer, so I said, "What's that?" I was told that the sonogram detected whether the lump was solid or liquid. That was all the caller said. I said to myself, "So what?" I was even more annoyed that I had to go back. I wondered why they kept bothering me. I was in good health. I practice Tai Chi daily. I didn't take any medications for anything. My blood pressure and cholesterol levels were normal. I even have all of my teeth at my age! I wanted them to go away so I could get on with my life. However, soon I received a telephone call to come in for a biopsy. Well, I knew what that meant. But since there is not a history of cancer in my family, I felt I had nothing to fear.

The doctor who performed the biopsy was an African-American female physician. She made me feel very comfortable. However, I didn't get any information about the higher incidence of cancer among African-American women. I never received any counseling during this experience. I had no idea that breast cancer was more prevalent in African-American women. The doctor didn't say anything about breast cancer and race, even though she was an African-America physician. She should have given me this kind of information.

It turned out that the lump was so small that she didn't get enough tissue the first time she went in so she had to do the procedure again. Several days later, she called and told me that she wished she had better news. The lump turned out to be cancerous. The good thing was that the lump was really very small indeed—so small, the doctor told me, she could have taken it out at the time of the biopsy. Amazed, I asked, "Well, why the heck didn't you?" She said that she was not allowed to do so. That really made me mad! I was still annoyed and not frightened, but I had a nagging feeling that perhaps the disease had spread.

I am a positive person who believes in a holistic approach to life. The doctor explained that surgery followed by chemotherapy was the best option. She also said they would test the lymph system to determine if the cancer had spread. I told her on the spot that I would not submit to chemotherapy. I didn't want my hair to fall out! I also did not want any changes in my lifestyle or to feel tired all the time. I quizzed her about radiation treatment. At home, I went on the Internet and looked up as much information about cancer and its treatment as I could find. I wanted to understand all I could about what was happening to me.

I knew that I had to tell my family at this point. Before that, I had gone through these kinds of experiences alone. I decided to tell just my daughters, my sisters, and several of my closest female friends. I told them the facts—that I had had a mammogram and a sonogram and that the doctor suggested surgery to remove a small lump that was found to be cancerous. I asked them for their prayers and told them the date of the surgery.

The general reaction of my family members was sorrow, dismay, and apprehension. The exception was my oldest daughter who is practical and down to earth like me. My youngest daughter registered shocked silence over the phone and very shortly flew in from Chicago—I live in Maryland—and accompanied me to my follow-up examinations.

Friends with whom I shared the news expressed concern and offered support. One friend, a member of SisterScribes, the writer's group that I host, helped me with errands and other things that I needed to do. I did speak to the cancer survivors among my friends and relatives. There were other friends and my brothers, with whom I did not share the information until after the surgery and after the report that the cancer had not spread. Even so, one of my co-workers looked at me with horror on his face and asked me if I was terrified. That wasn't very helpful. In fact, that really ticked me off! I told him to go away and pushed him away when he tried to give me a hug. I knew that he was concerned for me, but I didn't want any pity. I guess you might call me a feisty senior citizen!

I believe that my holistic lifestyle really helped me after surgery. I found strength in the application of "chi" meditation and prayer. However, something else upset me. After the surgery, the oncologist said that chemotherapy was not needed in my case. What would have happened if I had said "yes" to chemotherapy the first time it was suggested? However, I never would have done that. The oncologist did recommend a pill that you take twice daily. When she explained that the side effects might include osteoporosis, blood clots, and digestive problems, I would have none of that either.

This experience has been both eye-opening and tiring. But my attitude remains positive. This senior citizen has places to go and things to do and no time to be tired.

DR. RUTH KING

Lea

Lea Spencer, formerly the director of the Sacramento Black Chamber of Commerce, now manages security systems for a social work agency. The White doctors in her HMO called this professional Black woman "crazy" when she told them that there was something really wrong with her. After two years of misdiagnosis, a cancer research facility diagnosed her with leukemia and called her "the sickest patient" they had ever seen. And that's just the beginning of Lea's story of struggle and survival against difficult and heart-wrenching circumstances.

I am happy to write to you that I have survived leukemia for thirteen years. However, my journey has been a long and hard one. And, as you will see from this letter, this disease has decimated my family. It recently took the life of my only son at the age of twenty-nine and it has afflicted many other members of my family. But my story is about more than having a deadly disease and seeing loved ones suffer with it as well. My story begins with the negative attitudes of White doctors towards me.

I learned early that the worst position in this health care system is to be a sick Black woman, because most physicians don't believe what you tell them. Their attitude towards me delayed my treatment for two years. They made me even sicker.

Before my diagnosis, I was seen on a regular basis at an HMO. I had persistent flu-like symptoms and was often tired. I did everything that I could to get the HMO to find out what was wrong with me. I even went to the chief of medicine who gave me a call at home and pretty much said that I was a psychiatric case and that I needed to seek counseling.

I was very fortunate to get an appointment at a research medical facility at the University of California at Davis. Shortly thereafter, I was diagnosed with leukemia and started treatment within two hours of being seen. The doctors told me that I was the sickest patient they had ever treated and that they did not expect me to live through my treatment. That is why my recovery was so miraculous to them. What was not miraculous was my late diagnosis. The doctors at the HMO caused this to happen. They didn't listen to me, nor did they believe me, and they didn't follow up properly. To them I was some crazy Black woman who didn't want to go to work. I was living in Sacramento, which was extremely racist at that time. I had a doctor tell me, "You need to go back to work. You don't want to be like a dog with its tail between its legs and just run away from your job. Once you go back to work, you will feel better."

These kinds of comments stalled my treatment. But I continued to pursue finding out what was wrong with me. I filed complaints and changed doctors two or three times. However, once a doctor sees you and notes in your chart that "this person appears to have stress-related psychological issues," most doctors don't look past that. They just say, "Well, here she comes again." And that's what happened to me.

After I got well, I even tried to sue the HMO. But my lawyer made the point that I was still alive. Apparently, my legal case might have been more successful had I died!

When I went for my appointment at the research facility, I was feeling really bad. My throat was swollen because the cancer cells had attacked my lymph nodes. Fortunately, these doctors decided to do a blood test. That's when they found out that I had leukemia.

I received excellent care at the research facility. I became part of a clinical trial. The drugs worked. I had a lot of complications because I was diagnosed so late. But I am back working now in a new job.

My son's case was worse than mine. At a county hospital in Oakland, California, he was diagnosed with non-Hodgkin's lymphoma. He died within three months, after receiving what I would call very bad care. His condition and his death really took a lot out of me. I remember holding his hand in the hospital right before he died. I was just so tired.

My story doesn't end there. I found out that my family, my daughters, and my son in Sacramento were living in an area that is now being investigated as a cancer cluster. For almost a year and a half, *The Sacramento Bee* had reported the high incidents of leukemia and non-Hodgkin's lymphoma in the southern Sacramento neighborhood called Calvine-Florin—as much as 300 percent higher than in other areas in Sacramento. The State of California denies that there is anything unusual about the high incidence of these diseases and has put the burden on the neighborhood to prove that its residents live inside a cancer cluster. Recently, the *Bee* itself commissioned a study of the metal tungsten, an environmental contaminant, in the area's tree rings.

The debate goes on as to whether that area really is a cancer cluster or if these extremely high incidences of cancer are "coincidental." For me, it is silly to talk about coincidence. Maybe the state inspectors should move to the cancer cluster and see if they and their families get the disease.

I spoke to a *Sacramento Bee* reporter and he said that our family was unique. Of the 200 families that he had spoken with, we were the only household to have three family members diagnosed with cancer. My daughter has been diagnosed with pre-cancerous cells as well. I don't really know how we got these cancers, but it's my belief that we were contaminated by the tap water that we drank and the water that we swam in behind the house we lived in for nine years. At one time, a dry cleaning business was polluting the creek, and contaminants may have gotten into the water supply.

Even that's not the end of our family's battle with cancer. My husband's mother died of breast cancer six months after we were married. His stepmother also died of cancer. His sister was diagnosed with it and my husband's aunt has been diagnosed as well. My son was married and had three sons. Six months after they lost their dad, their grandmother died of cancer.

I think we as African Americans need to realize that doctors are just everyday people who have their own problems and prejudices. Just because you put on a white Lab coat doesn't mean that you now treat every patient fairly. When you go into a doctor's office, you don't know how White physicians feel about you as a person of color. There's nothing to say that they can remove their personal feelings from their work.

Most medical books have been written on a medical model that presupposes patients are White and male. Most drugs have been tested on White men and women. Just because it's medicine, doesn't erase the racism that's alive and well out there. My commitment is to try and have an impact on new physicians. With my involvement with the U.C. Davis Medical Center, I was able to work with the deans and a woman's health group and help them make physicians more aware of how to deal with patients of different cultures. I also did work with the Judy Davis Bone Marrow Group, which did a bone marrow drive for me. I tried to help get the word out into the African-American community about the need for bone marrow samples for possible matches for people of color.

Cancer is a terrible illness and not every one of us who gets it will come out alive. But a lot more African Americans *can* get out of it alive if we educate ourselves. We also need to have the strength and the courage to question our physicians and nurses and be persistent about advocating for ourselves.

My reality is that I truly hate cancer. This ugly disease just reared its head and now my family and I can't make it go away. For 13 years, cancer has been a scourge to my family and me. It affects us financially, emotionally, and spiritually. It truly makes me wonder what's going on. Why did God spare me and then take the life of my only son?

LEA SPENCER

Tom

Tom Jones is an advertising professional. A bit on the feisty side, Tom fought for the right to have good treatment for his colon cancer. Previously, he also listened to complete strangers who told him to get a colonoscopy. That may be why he's still here.

My story is probably a bit bizarre. Actually, it would even be funny if it were not I who went through it. When I walked into an Italian restaurant four years ago, I had no cancer symptoms whatsoever. While I was eating, the owner sat at my table to chat. For no reason at all, he told me that the previous day he had a colonoscopy. Now that I was over fifty, he said, I also should go get one. I said, "How do you know how old I am?" White people are notoriously bad about judging the age of Black people.

He said that when he was in Vietnam, he hung out with Black soldiers because the White soldiers were racist beyond his wildest imagination. That's why he knew how old I was. I didn't follow his advice. This was the first time that anyone had ever suggested having a colonoscopy to me. After all, what did he know anyway? About two weeks later, while I was standing in the checkout line at the health food store, another White guy, again out of the blue, told me I should have a colonoscopy. I thought to myself, what am I, a target for unsolicited advice from White guys who come out of nowhere to tell me about my health?

Starting around that time, I got a pain in my chest below the breastbone. I thought that it was indigestion. I took many different over-the-counter medicines, but the pain would not go away. It lasted close to a month.

Weirdly enough, just at that time I got a call from a gastroenterologist I had met a year earlier. His office called to ask me to come in about some medicine. This provided me with the opportunity to see the chief of gastroenterology at one of the best hospitals in Long Island. I told him about my pain and he said that he wanted to do an endoscopy to see if I had an ulcer. "Well," I said, "as long as I am out, why don't you do a colonoscopy? It's at the top of my mind now because two White guys I didn't know brought it up to me."

The next thing I knew, the surgeon woke me up and showed me photographs of two tumors in my colon the size of golf balls. He said that he couldn't tell whether or not they were cancerous, but that if they grew they could block off the opening to my small intestine. I would at that point be a very sick person. He told me I could come in later as an emergency patient and have an operation, or decide to do it now.

The nurses asked me how I knew to have this elective surgery. Again, I told them I had gotten a message from God in the form of two White guys I didn't know. What made it especially surprising is that cancer isn't the type of thing that men, Black *or* White, often talk about. You know, Norman Vincent Peale said that, "God works through coincidences." Well, he sure did on me.

A month later I had the operation, followed by a couple of months of convalescing. I was weak. I really wanted to go back to work, but my surgeon laughed at me. After two months, I went back to work but I got tired easily from chemotherapy.

My family was sympathetic but scared. No one had ever seen me in this kind of weakened condition before. To strengthen myself, I went out on little walks. But chemotherapy, no matter how you slice it, makes you weaker. My assessment is that chemo poisons you—but not enough to kill you, just enough to kill the cancer that's living inside you. When you are finished, your body does everything it can to expel these cells—you throw up, you sweat, you pee every 20 minutes, you have diarrhea, and your nose keeps running.

Gradually, I built up my strength. Three years later, I went to my regular doctor and found out that my white blood cell count was up again. So back to the gastroenterologist I went. I had a CAT scan, a PET scan and a CP PET scan for more detail. The last scan detected a growth on the outside of my colon.

The second operation went a lot better than the first. Three weeks later, I was ready to go back to work. I was better physically, but the process of having cancer twice debilitated me psychologically. Having parts of my colon cut out twice kind of got to me. A year later, uncomfortable with how weak I felt, I joined a gym. I am still alive and doing okay.

This experience with cancer taught me a few things about how to deal with a medical staff. My advice is to keep track of every procedure you have and every doctor that works on you. Not in a nasty way, just so that you know what they are doing to you. I'm a New Yorker, so this kind of thing comes naturally to me. I also have a lot of friends and relatives who helped me in this process. They would gripe about things that went wrong and the hospital staff set them right most of the time. Also, pay attention to your bill. Hospitals do make mistakes.

Even though I received excellent care, several mistakes *were* made in my case. I pointed out the mistakes—again, not in a nasty way. I told the hospital staff that my insurance pays the bills and that I pay my insurance. That means the hospital staff, all of them, work for me. They got the point.

You should also know that many of the people in the hospital who are responsible for your comfort are Black and Latino. So get to know them by name, respect them, and get them to take care of you. They really do want to do a good job for you.

The moral of my story is, don't let them treat you like a piece of meat. You are paying for this experience. Get what you pay for. Also, don't be rude. Just be firm. And don't let them write anything down without your knowing what it is they are putting into your file.

This experience has also taught me that life can be really fragile. I feel emotionally numb after all of this and I'm fighting a "what's the use" attitude. But I'm also thankful. Just by dumb luck, I found out that this disease was trying to kill me and I was able to stop it. So I guess the moral to my story is, get to know the surgeon who calls you a year after you first meet him and refers you to the chief of oncology at a world-class Jewish hospital on Long Island. And know that it is okay to listen to two White guys who don't know you but tell you to get a diagnostic procedure you don't think you need, or ever even heard of in the first place. You never know. God could be talking through them to you.

TOM JONES

Jim

Jim Wells is a well-known East Coast photographer and videographer. He has survived not only a bout with bladder cancer, but an aortic aneurysm as well. Jim can still be seen at the White House, on Capitol Hill and wherever the news is, camera clicking away. He also teaches photography at a local high school and a local college.

Life's a...well you know. But then you *don't* have to die. This is *not* thanks to my first urologist, who was Black by the way. I would like to punch him in the mouth but that won't do any good now. In my case, it wasn't the color of the person that mattered, it was his lack of experience...and mine too, I guess.

For a whole year tests showed that there were some anomalous cells in my bladder. I had a cystostomy and they found nothing. I had tests for a year and nothing more turned up, but I wasn't satisfied because I kept having discoloration in my urine. In a funny way, the fact that my first doctor was Black set me back. I trusted him more. But something told me that things weren't right.

I fired my first urologist and got someone—old, White and much more experienced—who was referred to me by a friend. This guy was the dean of urology at a respected institution and had worked on presidents and admirals. In a week, he found cancer in my bladder. Boy, was I pissed. (That's a urology joke!)

We had been working on this with the first urologist for an entire year and nothing was found. I believe that the cancer should have been detected much earlier. But I learned something, too. The first time around, I did not research the experience and capabilities of my doctor. The second time around, I did a research job and came up with the most experienced physician that I could find and that I could get a personal referral to. I began chemotherapy that lasted for about six months. Unfortunately, this did not reduce the size of the tumors. I believe that was because the first guy took too long and didn't detect the problem.

The bladder surgery came almost two years after they first suspected cancer and a year after I changed doctors. In between, I also had surgery when it was discovered that I had an aortic aneurysm. That was certainly one heck of a beginning to the new century! At first, I told only my wife and some immediate friends. I am in a business where perception is important. I just didn't feel the world had to know about my situation.

My wife's first reaction to the diagnosis was fear. We are all afraid of cancer, but she was probably more afraid than I was. I heard the diagnosis but I didn't totally accept it. I was also hopeful that chemotherapy or radiation would handle it without surgery. I didn't tell my daughters until after my operation. I didn't want to upset or involve them.

To this day, I am not really sure what caused the cancer. In my case, it could have been any number of things. I have been a professional photographer for nearly forty years. We handled a lot of chemicals in the old days. At that time, we didn't use gloves and masks. We also used powdered chemicals instead of liquids, so the stuff got into the air. Sometimes the ventilation wasn't that good either. I have also done photographic assignments on location in military facilities. In some cases, we had film fogged from as much as a half mile away. I don't know why. My cancer also could have come about from my days in the Air Force. I was working on B-52 Bombers and my job was to work with bombing navigation gear and I sometimes worked with atomic bombs. I also worked with the wave guides for radar and with a lot of other nuclear devices as well.

In the late 1950s, we didn't know very much about shielding, so who knows what happened? Although we had Geiger counters, we didn't have the sophisticated testing devices that there are today. However, I do count myself lucky. I really don't operate much differently than I did before. I am more consistent about going to the doctor and getting check-ups to make sure that nothing else occurs. My biggest fear is that I will get another form of cancer. I did smoke cigarettes for a long while. Obviously, I've stopped now and I haven't been diagnosed with lung cancer. So far, so good, knock on wood.

I wasn't in much pain from the bladder cancer procedures. But the aortic aneurysm operation was the most painful event of my life. It made me 96 years old in 24 hours. I had to have this surgery before the bladder operation and it held up my cancer procedure for at least four months. But again, I count myself lucky. I had good support systems. My wife and friends really helped me. Since I am a photographer, I have to carry around a lot of equipment. During my recovery, I could not have done that without the help of some of the guys who I got into the business and a good friend who is an architect. My friends came with me on my photo assignments to make sure that I didn't overdo it physically. One friend had his daughter, who is a nurse, come over and assist me. This is funny, but even my dog helped. Before the surgery, he was nicer to me than he usually is; he often came and sat by my feet. I think that he knew something was wrong. Now, of course, he just wants his food and to go for a walk.

I guess I should have listened to a friend of mine, who was at the time, president of the National Association of Urologists. He told me to get tested, but I took him too lightly. I should have listened to him and gotten tested earlier. That really would have helped.

JIM WELLS

CHAPTER SIX

It's All in the Family

WE ARE CAUGHT IN AN INESCAPABLE NETWORK OF
MUTUALITY, TIED IN A SINGLE GARMENT OF DESTINY.
WHATEVER AFFECTS ONE DIRECTLY AFFECTS ALL
INDIRECTLY. AS LONG AS THERE IS POVERTY IN THIS
WORLD, NO MAN CAN BE TOTALLY RICH EVEN IF HE
HAS A BILLION DOLLARS. AS LONG AS DISEASES ARE
RAMPANT AND MILLIONS OF PEOPLE CANNOT EXPECT
TO LIVE MORE THAN TWENTY OR THIRTY YEARS, NO
MAN CAN BE TOTALLY HEALTHY, EVEN IF HE JUST GOT
A CLEAN BILL OF HEALTH FROM THE FINEST CLINIC IN
AMERICA.

—Martin Luther King, Jr., *I Have a Dream*

Elizabeth

Elizabeth's bout with cancer was not a solitary ordeal. Her mother was diagnosed and died while Elizabeth was still in treatment. What kept Elizabeth going was the loving support of her family, which she returned by educating them about prevention and early treatment of cancer.

Retirement was the beginning of a new plateau in my life, which had all the allure and excitement I dreamed it would. I had just returned from a 16-day Mediterranean cruise. Traveling is a passion I could now enjoy to the fullest.

Then my bubble burst. Two weeks after my return in November, 2001, my annual mammogram showed that I had breast cancer. I went from jubilation to speculation and fear. Cancer is a family matter. So my two grown sons and a daughter-in-law went with me to doctor appointments, aided me in making decisions, and supported me with an outpouring of love. We all did a lot of research and then met to discuss the different options I had. Fortunately my son, Jason Murray, is in pharmaceutical sales and his wife, Tanya, is a registered nurse; they were able to find invaluable information that ultimately led me to my selection of a surgeon, medical oncologist, and radiation oncologist.

My other son, Desmond Murray, assistant director of field experience, and affirmative action officer of Marist College, shared the news of my condition with a woman he knew who recently had been diagnosed with the same aliment. She constantly communicated with me and led me through the process, calming much of my fear.

Blessings unfolded when, in January 2002, I was afforded the latest technology in the medical field during the preparation and execution of my surgery. Locating the tumor in the early stage put me in a category for best chances of survival. The FDA had just approved Arimidex™, a medication given to breast cancer patients, including those in early stages. Previous to that, Arimidex™ was only prescribed for advanced cancer patients.

Once you have breast cancer you always have a chance of recurrence, so every decision you make is an attempt to increase your life span. This is where I rely on my religious faith and my belief in the Almighty to guide my choices.

My family was not only faced with my diagnosis, but at the same time my 86-year-old mother became sick with bladder cancer and was hospitalized for four months. Two days after her admittance, I began my postoperative radiation treatments in the same hospital, even though my surgery had been performed in a different one. Because of nurse understaffing, I was blessed again in that I was able to spend mornings and afternoons assisting with my mother's care.

God gave me the strength and stamina to spend a great deal of quality time with my mom but, because she needed 24-hour care, three days before my radiation treatments were over she was transferred to Calvary Hospital in the Bronx, N.Y., one of the most renowned cancer hospice facilities in the United States. She ultimately graduated to glory 54 days later. In my mourning, I saw clearly how precious life is and how hard I have to fight for my own survival.

Overall, my life has been enriched by the many opportunities I have been offered, even through times of suffering. I've met so many positive people and, with their help, I've learned and adopted healthier ways of eating. In addition, I've increased my self-esteem and well-being. I have been a survivor for almost two years now. During that time, I have faced many obstacles. For instance, I love dancing, but the radiation and the medication made me so exhausted that I was unable to complete a three-minute dance. Now I'm just about back to normal. Besides dancing, I bowl in two leagues and am even traveling again.

I consider myself cancer-free, but cancer is never far from my mind. I participate weekly in a cancer support group as well as a clinical yoga study session for breast cancer survivors held at Einstein Hospital in the Bronx. My sons and I participated in the Susan G. Komen Walk for the Cure in September 2003, in Central Park in Manhattan.

I have also been a vocal advocate for breast cancer awareness whenever I get an opportunity. After I was diagnosed, I contacted my sisters and other relatives asking them to make appointments for mammograms. My own diagnosis placed my siblings in a high-risk category for developing cancer.

Cancer is a family matter. You need the support of loved ones in making decisions about your choice of treatment and about who will be performing that treatment. It is very important to be extremely diligent about check-ups and to communicate well with your physician.

Last month, my brother informed me that he has been diagnosed with prostate cancer (early stage). He and his doctor have been watching his PSA numbers. Our family has come together again to support him and thus ensure the best possible recovery from his ordeal. We are supportive of each other spiritually and understand the power of a strong family network.

ELIZABETH B. MURRAY

Tina

Tina, a breast cancer survivor, is originally from Zaire. Her grandfather and father died of prostate cancer. She hopes that Americans will come to help cancer victims in countries that don't presently have the technology and the medicines to successfully treat them.

Although I am originally from Zaire, I was diagnosed with breast cancer while living in Washington, D.C. I discovered the abnormality in my left breast myself. I am a medical doctor, so I had several advantages over the average woman in my native country.

One night after my shower, I noticed something unusual in the mirror so I conducted a breast self-exam. While conducting the exam, everything I learned in medical school about breast cancer came into my memory. It was in the upper outer quadrant of my left breast (one of the worst places a woman can find a lump). I was sure that something was wrong so I contacted an oncologist. He stated that I was under stress and to ignore it, but I could not ignore it. Nobody listened to my concerns because I did not fit the profile of someone who would get cancer. I am athletic. I do not smoke and drink only occasionally. I eat healthy meals and I am not overweight. In addition, I am under 40 years of age with three kids. The only positive factor was indeed the stress that almost everybody experiences here in the U.S.

Three months later, after my workout at the gym, I felt hard bumps in my left underarm. I requested my oncologist friend to set an appointment for me. Two mammograms did not show cancer, but the radiologist insisted that I have another exam. I had an ultrasound that indicated cancer.

My cancer was diagnosed at Stage IIB. Thank God I insisted on being examined, because cancer had started in the right breast too. Eventually I had a double mastectomy and lymph node removal. The entire process took place in three surgeries within six weeks. Then I went through seven months of chemotherapy and began taking Tamoxifen™.

It is difficult to describe the pain and suffering of chemotherapy. It is really hell! I was devastated to be a cancer victim. For more than a year, I was in denial and refused to wear prostheses. Now I am over it.

My family does not talk about cancer at all, but unfortunately cancer is common in Zaire. Prostate cancer is especially common. My paternal grandfather died of prostate cancer at age 69 and my dad, although a medical doctor, also died of prostate cancer at age 69. Thyroid cancer and liver cancer are also common.

Some myths in my country prevent early detection. Only two to three decades ago, it was a general belief that African-American people did not suffer from cancer, only White people did. Now with more people receiving education and more families having loved ones die of this disease, many of these false statements are no longer believed.

Few people in Zaire know to recognize the first symptoms. If they did, they could catch the cancer at an early stage. Even then, they would face a problem. Few of our hospitals are equipped with the kinds of high technology equipment that help in early diagnosis, especially of cancers like cervical or breast cancer. Many clinicians are obliged to rely on physical signs and symptoms.

Unhappily, for these reasons cancer is considered a death sentence for most people in my country. Nobody wants to mention that word or to even think about it. Wealthy people go to South Africa for treatment, since it is one of the few countries in Africa with the kind of diagnostic techniques and medicine that may slow and ultimately even cure cancer.

That is why I pray that Americans become sensitive to the needs of people in other countries concerning the care and successful treatment of cancer.

TINA MBOYAMBA

Don

Don Williford was a tough man, with two tours of Vietnam and a thirty-year career in the U.S. Army under his belt. That didn't keep prostate cancer from striking him. But, mental toughness and discipline did help him not only survive, but thrive. He now helps others as a facilitator of a prostate awareness group at Walter Reed Hospital in Washington, D.C.

As I grew up in suburban Philadelphia, the fact that I was adopted wasn't talked about. Later, when I needed a birth certificate to register for ROTC at Temple University, I was shocked to find out that I was adopted. One of my major missions in life was to meet my biological father.

After a lot of looking, I met my biological father in 1982 and spent ten great years with him. He died of prostate cancer just prior to his 85th birthday in July 1992. My father had refused chemotherapy and radiation treatment. He didn't want anything. My father never talked about cancer. He didn't want anyone to know he had the disease. By the time of my father's death, I'd already started learning what I could about cancer.

When my father got very ill, I had a hard time knowing what to do when I sat at his bedside or nursed him. My college advisor told me to let my father do the talking. But my father never did.

After my father died, I read about the disease for almost a decade and had yearly check-ups, assuming I would also have to face prostate cancer. My PSA numbers first went outside the window in 1995; I had three biopsies between 1995 and 1998 without detection of cancer. In August of 2000, my PSA was elevated to eighteen and cancer cells were detected.

My doctor and I had a conversation and I told him I wanted surgery. The point is to get the cancer out. The surgeons look at the adjacent tissues and send them to the pathologist while you are open. If there is cancer in the adjacent tissues, then they have to do some more cutting. The neurovascular bundles on each side of the prostate control a man's ability to have an erection. I said to check the bundles and if they were diseased, take them out. I don't care about an erection. I want to live. I had successful surgery on November 30, 2000, and I take no medication. With Viagra, I am fully functional.

I opted for surgery because I'm not the kind of guy who wants to live with a time bomb inside me. Radiation may not get it all. It's a crapshoot. My first choice was to get rid of all of the cancer.

I now facilitate the Prostate Cancer Awareness Group at Walter Reed Hospital. The hospital folks were going to kill the outreach group at Walter Reed because of poor attendance. I said no. I have a responsibility to my son and others coming behind us. Somebody said that the board had to make a decision and I said, "Damn the board. I will be here. Who will be here with me?" Eventually, I was asked to be the facilitator.

We're there to support each other and to provide laymen's answers to the questions of those who are newly diagnosed, who are like deer in the headlights. They are scared. They think that they are going to die next week. The group is up to twenty-six people per month and people come from as far away as North Carolina and Connecticut. We take the disease seriously, but we don't take ourselves too seriously.

I am really concerned that many African-American men have the attitude that removal of the prostate will mess with their sexuality. They think, "I'm not a man anymore if I get this disease." That negativity is what kills many of us. We also have to get over our fear.

We have a mobile van that does prostate cancer screening and testing. We went down to a mall in D.C. For nearly half an hour, I tried to convince one guy to get tested. He was 37 years old, had two children, and his father had died of prostate cancer. He did not want to go into the van. Finally I said, "Do you love your wife and children?" He said, "Yes." He finally admitted that he was scared. He asked me to go into the van with him. I went in with him and he got his exam. His results, of course, were confidential. This kind of personal touch exemplifies my approach to helping African-American men in the Washington, D.C. area.

Everyone needs to know that someone cares. It is also important to gain insight from those who have been there before. We do both and provide accurate information as well.

DON WILLIFORD

JEROLINE

Jeroline's physician ignored the signs of cancer. She got rid of that doctor but continued having troubling health concerns. The second doctor she went to discovered that she had colon cancer. Jeroline survived, but cancer continues to plague her family. During her struggle, she lost her mother to colon cancer. More recently, both her father and her brother were diagnosed with the same cancer. With her friends, family and her strong faith to support her, Jeroline remains positive about her life and her future.

The first doctor I went to when I knew my body wasn't working right told me that I wasn't old enough to have colon cancer. Today, as a twenty-two-year cancer survivor, when I think about that doctor's carelessness, I can only shake my head. For a year he treated me for hemorrhoids because I had blood in my stool. I followed his recommendations for a whole year, I'm sorry to say. Only when I saw that I wasn't getting any better did I change doctors.

My new doctor sent me to the hospital for a colonoscopy. A few days later, she called me at work to say that she good news and bad news. I said, "Give me the bad news first." When she told me that I had colon cancer, I dropped the phone and started crying uncontrollably. A friend in the office came out to see if I was alright. Finally, I composed myself long enough to ask the doctor for the good news. My cancer was operable, he told me, and then he scheduled me for surgery the following week.

Before I went to the hospital for surgery, my doctor told me I might have to wear a colostomy bag for the rest of my life. At first I said I would rather die and I refused to have the surgery. At that time, I was afraid to tell my friends that I had cancer. I was not sure how they would handle the news. Eventually, I shared my diagnosis with people close to me. They were very supportive and told me that I should trust in God and have the surgery. So I did and it was successful.

I am still self-conscious about the very large scar that resulted from the surgery, but that scar, like the emotional ones, is slowly healing. I've learned from this experience that nothing is too hard for God. With that support, I also learned to take a positive attitude about life no matter how bad things look.

I weighed about 100 pounds before the surgery and my medical team had to "build me up" before the operation. With their help, I was able to bring my body up to the ordeal of surgery. The first thing I heard when I woke up from surgery was my doctor saying that I did not have to wear a colostomy bag. There was more good news. Instead of removing my entire colon, they took out eighteen inches and were able to reconnect the colon. My doctor told me that my recovery period would be approximately seven to ten days. I went home on the third day to complete my recovery there.

Just before I left the hospital, I was advised to have a colonoscopy every six months for a year, then once a year, and now every five years. I had my last colonoscopy just a few months ago and there are no signs of cancer.

That is not the end of my story. Just two years after my own battle with cancer, my mother was diagnosed with colon cancer. By the time they discovered her cancer, the disease had already spread to other organs of her body and it was too late. She lived about nine months after her diagnosis. My mother really suffered before she died and that tore me apart. I had a nervous breakdown just watching the mother I loved so dearly die such a horrible death.

After my mother died, my dad was diagnosed with prostate cancer. He was treated and has recovered. Later, he was diagnosed with colon cancer. He had surgery and he is still surviving. Last year, my youngest brother was diagnosed with colon cancer. He has been treated now and is doing well. My positive attitude and faith in God have seen me through my own cancer and have helped me help my family members as well.

JEROLINE WALKER

Ramona

Ramona lost her sister and mother to cancer. That's why she insisted on receiving adequate cancer screening. Eventually, Ramona was diagnosed with lung cancer. Unlike her loved ones, Ramona survived to tell her story and it's a story she believes will help others. At the start of her ordeal, Ramona saw herself as a victim. Now she says with pride, "I am a survivor."

From 1972 to 2003, six of my family members, two special friends, and I were all diagnosed with some form of breast, stomach, cervical, or lung cancer. Two have survived, including myself.

For me, it started in September of 2000. I was doing something easy, like sweeping the floor, when I recognized that I felt really tired and that I had a burning sensation behind my right breast that felt like someone was pressing a hot glue gun there. No matter whether I was walking or sitting or lying, I couldn't escape the constant pain and no over-the-counter medication relieved it.

After I lost my mother and my sister to cancer, the grief I felt moved through my body like venom. But that emotional pain would give way to an unbearable physical pain. I was hesitant to find the source of this pain because I was without health insurance and I was afraid of the truth that awaited me. Like so many others, I hoped the problem would go away.

When it did not go away, I located an agency that provided free mammograms. I had one, but the doctor said there was no sign of any problems. I had several other consultations with health providers in that agency who came to the same conclusion: nothing was wrong with me. I now realize that most agencies that offer free services to minorities have very limited resources and usually are not technically equipped to detect serious problems. My agency didn't encourage me to get further testing. In a nutshell, for me these free services were a dangerous waste of time. My symptoms progressed and my frustrations grew. But I'd seen too many people close to me die because they were never properly tested. I know my body and my instincts told me something was not right. I decided to get the proper tests.

The next month consisted of X-rays, CAT scans, an MRI, and a breathing test. It wasn't an easy time, but I found some relief in knowing that once the doctors found out what was wrong, I could move to the next step—successful treatment. While I sat in waiting rooms, I sometimes cried for all my relatives and friends who had died of cancer. I cried for the strangers in the waiting room with me. Then, when I thought there were no more tears to shed, I cried for me.

Several specialists spoke with me on the day the results came back. The consensus was that there was a spot on my right lung that might be cancerous and might not. For reasons I cannot explain, when I heard this news I began polishing my nails. I guess I did it because it was a routine that required my concentration and it stopped the shaking. When one of the doctors returned to find me polishing my nails, she said this was a reaction she had never seen before. As my nails dried, we both found a moment to smile.

On July 31, 2001, the day of my surgery, my daughter and I arrived at 7 a.m. and checked in with the nurse who prepared me for the operation. As I sat in my hospital gown, I glanced at my daughter sitting across from me with this worried and frightened look on her face. We were both overcome with fear, heartache, and tears. We cried for the things we had said to one another and the things we had not. As we embraced, we expressed love, both spoken and unspoken, like only a mother and daughter can comprehend. Then I said, "See you shortly."

About seven hours later, I found myself sitting in a chair in front of my daughter and there was my brother, standing in the doorway. A nurse said, "Can you tell me your name?" "Ramona," I told her, even though I was still a bit wobbly from the medication. "And how old are you, Ramona?" she asked again. "Thirty-seven," I said. "She's forty-three!" my daughter quickly corrected, then added, "She's okay, nurse. She does that all the time."

I was alive and well. Soon my oldest and dearest friends came to see me. I remember saying how beautiful everyone looked. I had survived. I did a lot of praying before, during, and after my tribulations. I didn't make any special requests. I just let God know that I trusted His will. In my heart I knew that my own situation was so very small compared to the emotional stress of losing my mother and my sister. However, I had survived to realize the importance of my story as a survivor of the disease.

I continue to look for God's purpose in sparing my life. At the start of this ordeal, I saw myself as a victim. Then God sent people to help me see that I am a survivor. As I breathe through two healthy lungs, I pray that my story offers someone encouragement, faith and hope.

RAMONA CROSS

Dolly

There was a history of fibrocystic disease in Dolly's family, so she did not panic when she first felt a lump in her breast. She assumed that it was fibrocystic disease. Years later, she was diagnosed with breast cancer. With the help of family members, friends, and her church, Dolly was able to endure treatment. She thanks God for helping her deal with the diagnosis.

I was 49 years old when I felt the first lump in my breast. I am one of many women in my family who have fibrocystic disease, so I did not believe I had a serious illness. My doctor did a biopsy and the test came back negative. Then one day, while in my laundry room, my right breast brushed against the wall and I felt a slight pain. Later, I conducted a breast self-examination and found a lump. I called my doctor's office again and went in for an exam.

This time my doctor conducted a needle aspiration. We found that the lump was not filled with fluid as before, but solid. I knew then that I had a problem. My doctor decided to do a second biopsy. There would be many more. It took a while before I decided to tell my family the results of the tests, because I knew there were more to come—the next one surgical.

While I waited to go into surgery, my nurse explained that the doctor would be taking a sample of the tissue in the lump and around it as well. Three days later, when I went in alone as usual to get the results, the nurse sent for my husband. Then the doctor told both of us that I had breast cancer and that I would need additional surgery. I decided to have a lumpectomy instead of a mastectomy. I knew how lucky I was and I thanked God. Out of the four stages of cancer, I had the first stage—the least dangerous.

My husband and I called our families. Because they did not hear fear in my voice, they were encouraged. Family and friends rallied around us, and my sisters came in from out of town for my surgery. I had a lumpectomy and the surgeon also removed one lymph node. When I woke up from surgery, my family and friends were there waiting. I was in a lot of pain, but I was alive.

My cancer was an aggressive kind but, because I found it early, the cancer had not spread beyond the breast. After I recovered from surgery, I went to see an oncologist, who prescribed six months of chemotherapy and 31 days of radiation. He said that I might not get sick or lose my hair, but I *did* get sick, and I did lose my hair.

God had some lessons for me to learn. I am the type of person who would do everything I could for others, but it's hard for me to accept help. Over the next six months I would need a lot of help.

A month after surgery I started my chemo treatments. The first couple of months I was fine. But then I began to feel the side effects, and it took me a while to recover from the treatments. I have a high threshold for pain, but I found it hard to handle the sick feeling I got from chemo. I dreaded each treatment.

I cannot tell you how important phone calls, cards, and words of encouragement were to me. I received a lot, and I thank God for them all. The deacon at my church was especially helpful. He also had cancer and he gave me some good suggestions about things to get me through the treatment. For example, he said sucking on popsicles would keep me from feeling sick and he told me to use baking soda to rinse my mouth so as not to get mouth sores. I did both and they worked, so I passed the tips on to other cancer patients.

I eventually began radiation treatments. I remember the day: it was February of 1997 and it was a mild winter. I had to go to Akron Hospital every weekday for 31 days. After chemo, radiation was not bad at all. Many people offered me rides and just their offering meant a lot to me.

Throughout my treatment, I continued to work. At first I missed a couple of days a month, and later, I missed a couple of weeks each month. Everyone at work was sympathetic to what I was going through and gave me their full support.

In the middle of my treatments, my husband, being very optimistic, booked a seven-day cruise to the Caribbean. This was to be my reward, and it gave me hope and something to focus on. We went on that cruise in October 1997 and had a great time.

God has truly provided the right people to care for me.

DOLLY LOWE

CHAPTER SEVEN

Healing:
Mind, Body and Spirit

HUMOR MAY NOT BE LAUGHTER, IT MAY NOT EVEN BE
A SMILE; IT IS A POINT OF VIEW, AN ATTITUDE
TOWARD AN EXPERIENCE.

—Howard Thurman, *Meditations of the Heart*

WHEN YOU GET INTO A FIGHT WITH A BEAR, YOU
DON'T GET TIRED UNTIL THE BEAR GETS TIRED.

—Coleman Young, *Detroit Free Press*

Barbara

Barbara's world turned upside down after her breast cancer diagnosis. She kept asking, "Why me?" because she didn't smoke or drink. That didn't change the diagnosis. Now after thirty-three radiation treatments, the only place she wants to see her doctor (after she is finally declared cancer-free) is at the shopping mall.

In 1994, calcifications were found in my breast during a routine, yearly mammogram. An incision biopsy confirmed that I had breast cancer. I left school during my lunch hour to discuss the findings of the biopsy. I was really scared, but trying to act like a big girl. After I was told that I had cancer and would need a partial mastectomy and axillary dissection, I got in my car and lost it. My crying came not from anger but from fear of the unknown.

On September 26th of that year, I had surgery and stayed in the hospital overnight. I was discharged with a drainage tube and given a prescription for antibiotics. The drainage tube remained until October 4th; another antibiotic was prescribed because of continued seepage. My surgical scar looks like a big, twisted smile. Following consultation with the radiation oncologist on October 11th, I returned on October 21st for markings to guide the oncologist during treatment. Radiation therapy began on October 24th.

On the following day, I joined an African-American cancer support group and found it to be an invaluable resource of kindred spirits. On October 27th, I met with the medical oncologist who explained to me that my tumor was 1.4 cm and very aggressive. I would need chemotherapy, two weeks on and two weeks off, for six months. The chemotherapy included Methotrexate, Fluorouracil, and Cyclophosphamide. Anti-nausea medications prescribed were Decadron,™ Zofran™ and Reglan.™

I began a cancer journal. On November 11, 1994, my journal entry read, "I will be on radiation and chemo at the same time. People think I'm sick. I'm not sick, I'm fighting to live. The cancer didn't hurt. What will all this stuff (medication and radiation) do to my body?"

The most overwhelming effect was fatigue. During a trip to the supermarket, I approached a gentleman sitting on a two-seated bench and remarked, "I am so tired that if that seat next to you belongs to someone else, I'll have to sit on your lap, sir."

Chemotherapy robbed me of self-control. I recall several incidents that left me feeling helpless. I found it important to be able to laugh at myself. That laughter helped me to gain the strength I needed to pull through. For example, I got up one morning and, because of fatigue, sat on the toilet for an hour. I realized I couldn't stay on the toilet all day. From that point on, I carried my cell phone with me everywhere. My belief in God and my own laughter helped me gain the strength that I needed to pull through all of the challenging times.

This experience has taught me there is a blessing in being able to share, a blessing in continued healing, a blessing of leaving a legacy as I live and heal, and a blessing of knowing that God is in my life. Cancer has made me a stronger person and I have had the blessing of being able to bond with so many strong women. I like to think of myself as a strong, dedicated survivor.

My goal in life has become advocacy for cancer education and early detection. I have a deep-rooted passion for dispelling the fear connected with cancer, and ending the silence that seems to surround the word "cancer." It is of the utmost importance for me to embrace many communities by educating as many individuals as possible.

BARBARA J. BECKWITH

Survivors

Survivors are proud of themselves. They respect themselves and others.

They are aware of who they are. They neither seek definition from the person they are with, nor expect them to read their minds. They are quite capable of articulating their needs.

Survivors are hopeful. They are strong enough to make all of their dreams come true. They know love; therefore, they give love. They recognize that their love has great value and must be reciprocated. If their love is taken for granted, it soon disappears.

Survivors have a dash of inspiration and a dab of endurance. They know that, at times, they will have to inspire others to reach the potential God gave them.

Survivors know their past, understand their present, and move toward their future with gusto.

Survivors know God. They know that with God the world is their playground, but without God they will just be played with.

Survivors do not live in fear of the future because of their past. Instead, they understand that their life experiences are merely lessons, meant to bring them closer to self-knowledge and unconditional love.

Barbara J. Beckwith

Ron

Ron grew up in the Baptist Church. Diagnosed with stomach cancer after he believed he had an ulcer, Ron approached every day as a blessing and walked in faith as he dealt with the cancer growing inside of him.

My lifelong faith has supported me during each moment of the past year. My family and friends have visited and prayed with me. I am blessed with excellent doctors and treatment. I appreciate the opportunity to share my story with you.

This journey has awakened me to every nuance of my physiology. I am about to undergo another operation brought on by my own observation of my body and with my insistence. My lifelong faith has supported me each moment along the way. I grew up in the Baptist Church and have maintained an active faith as an adult. That faith is what is seeing me through what has turned out to be a harrowing ordeal.

I was ill for three months with what I self-diagnosed as ulcers. I couldn't keep any food down. The physician I consulted diagnosed me with stomach cancer and said he wished I had come in sooner. I knew I would need a strong support system to get through this process so I told my family and friends about my illness right away. Shortly after my forty-seventh birthday, the doctors removed my stomach and I underwent radiation treatment following the operation. I had trouble with elimination and again was unable to keep down any nourishment.

Twenty-five days of radiation started to "cook" the scar tissue and caused my bowels to lock up. I re-entered the hospital, where the doctors ran a battery of tests with no results. The doctor who did the first operation performed a second one that showed many cancer tumors; he closed me up. One member of the team of surgeons suggested that I enter a hospice treatment program, but I thought I was too young to give up on my life, so I sought another medical opinion. Another brilliant physician devised a way to re-route the intestines around the blockage and operated again. The operation was a success and I began doing different kinds of rehab so that I could leave the hospital. But I felt another blockage, which turned out to be in the lower intestine. I'm going back into surgery next Monday.

My 90-year-old grandmother recently stayed three nights with me in the hospital. Her visit was so precious. This experience has shown me what I need to take care of and have in order, the importance of "keeping it real" because tomorrow is not promised, and to mend broken fences and resolve troubling relationships. I think I have worked steadily toward a resolution within myself, but I could not have come this far without the unwavering support of friends and family, and my faith in God.

Ronald L. Jones succumbed to cancer on February 2, 2004. He was 48.

Michelle

Michelle, a 10-year survivor of inflammatory breast cancer, proudly says, "Here I am." Her strong faith, together with using both conventional medicine and alternative remedies, has gotten her through a monumental challenge. She has recently taken on another challenge and entered law school.

Here I Am
I beat the odds that man had set for me. It has been ten years since I was diagnosed with Stage IV inflammatory breast cancer.

The survival rate is three percent and only six years. Well, it just goes to show you that even though doctors have a God-given talent to set up your healing, it is your faith in God that brings about the continued healing.

I have never asked myself why, because I know that God has miraculous healing power. My healing has been mind, body, and spirit. I never accepted the word "terminal." My faith in God, along with the power of reading His word and the health journals, gave me comfort. I used herbal remedies along with the pharmaceutical cocktails the doctors came up with. Cancer therapy is a lot of trial and error, but I do know that the most important part of the formula is faith—and the will to fight.

Since my diagnosis, I have inspired other cancer patients to fight to live. I believe that cancer will follow you wherever you go—face it, because you can't run from it. If you do, it runs with you, it becomes more powerful, and it will knock you down and take you out. My best advice is that you stand up and take it on. I was 39-years-old when cancer attempted to take me down. I am now 49-years-old and I am studying law.

When it's all said and done, I call it all joy. To God is the glory. Peace.

MICHELLE WILLIAMS

Grace

Like many others, Grace was misdiagnosed at first. But she made her traumatic experience work for her and beat the odds by surviving. Her strong faith helped her find a new mission in life—helping others by forming a non-profit organization that provides cancer education to those with little or no health insurance.

For about eight months, I had been ailing. My complaint was nondescript. I would wake up in the middle of the night with a "sick" feeling in my stomach. I would run to the bathroom, but my body did nothing in response. Going back to bed, I would lie awake and wonder.

My doctor examined me, ordered tests and wrote prescriptions. She thought I was having panic attacks. Finally, I told her that the episodes, lack of sleep, and anxiety were making me depressed. This time, I left with a prescription for Zoloft, an anti-depressant.

Three weeks later, on a Saturday morning, I had excruciating pain in my lower right side. I could not lift my legs to put on my underwear or my panty hose. When I tried to, the dead weight made me want to scream and I had to lift my leg with my hands. Driving my car was equally difficult. Lifting my foot from the brake to the accelerator nearly made me cry. By Wednesday evening, I was bawling.

At daybreak on Thursday morning, my daughter, Olethia, arrived with one of her church members, Mother Graves; the two of them insisted that I go to the emergency room. I was admitted. All day Thursday, Friday, and Saturday, I received tests, tests, and more tests, along with medication to kill the pain. I had had nothing by mouth since the Wednesday prior to being admitted to the hospital.

On Sunday evening, the gastroenterologist came to my bedside and said, "I've got good news for you. We have not found anything and since you no longer are in pain we are going to send you home tomorrow morning." The pain had subsided because of the pain medication.

I should have been glad to get the "good news" but I was not, because I was convinced something was wrong with me and they simply had not found it. When I returned to the doctor, Father God intervened and used my voice to reply. This is what he said through me: "You have looked at one-third of my colon. I think you need to look at my entire colon."

For four days, I had had nothing by mouth. Each of the tests came with all sorts of preparation, injections, and stuff to drink. By Sunday evening, I was quite weak from it all. I am not a physician—I hardly know where the colon is located—and I certainly didn't know the anatomy of the body well enough to understand that the focus of my discomfort was the colon.

But, to appease me, the gastroenterologist mentioned two different procedures—the sigmoidoscopy and the colonoscopy. I asked, "Which is the most precise?" He replied, "The colonoscopy." "Then, that's what I want," I told him.

The colonoscopy was done on Monday morning. I recall being semi-sedated, viewing the TV monitor, and hearing the doctor say, "Let's go back there. Let's look at that again." The finding: a cancerous tumor and villous cells in my cecum ("What in the world is a cecum?" I wondered). Monday night the surgeon was at my bedside and Tuesday morning I had major surgery—an extended right hemicolectomy.

There was little time for me to "feel" anything except exhilaration. No, I was not overjoyed that cancer was found in my body with metastasis to my lymph system. I was overjoyed that someone could now acknowledge my sanity and see that there was something wrong with me. Things happened very quickly. On Wednesday I was at work, Thursday I was in the hospital, on Monday I was diagnosed with cancer, and by Tuesday my life had been changed forever. My journey with cancer had begun.

During this journey, I began to have feelings about this diagnosis and its consequences. The impact hit me after I was alone at home recovering from surgery, dealing with my thoughts. As we all know, a diagnosis of cancer can send a person and that person's loved ones into a tailspin. "Oh God, it's cancer! What is going to happen to me? How long will I survive?" The diagnosis conjured up a multitude of emotions—fear, despair, depression, uncertainty, fatalism—all of which had a profound impact on me and on my loved ones. What does one do when told one has cancer? Where does one go for medical advice, emotional sustenance, and spiritual guidance?

Often the most probing questions are, "How long do I have to live? What is the prognosis? Am I going to die?" And on and on. There were far more questions than answers. In my mind, there were two courses that I could choose (and probably many more). I might simply go "limp" and virtually assume a position of doom and gloom or I could take flight and fight. I was ill-prepared to accept the diagnosis, but I was not prepared to go limp and give up. I considered the implications and contemplated a future, during this momentary confusion over what should be done. No matter what my response, I knew my life had been changed forever.

Suddenly, in the eyes of my healthcare providers I became just another patient under their care—Patient No. 123432 to be exact. But to me I was the person I had always known myself to be. You might wonder what I mean? Here is a partial list of descriptors—one as Patient, the other as Person.

As Patient No. 123432 I represented and/or required: hospitalization, vital signs, blood work, injections, meds/dosages, bandages, tests, X-rays, bone scans, imaging, examinations, treatments, consultations, bedpans—uck, mini-baths, chemotherapy, catheter, and on and on.

As Person, Grace Lillian Butler, I represented qualities that were suddenly under attack: needs, hopes, fears, attitudes, motivations, interests, dreams, likes/dislikes, relationships, careers, and most of all, spirituality. Obviously, each characteristic on the list of descriptors could be much longer. But the point is made: the person I had been was now subservient to the patient I had become. Certainly, the patient-related items were vitally important, but so were the others. I still saw myself as the person I had always known.

I know that healthcare providers, by and large, are trained to address the patient-related needs. As a patient, I appreciated that. However, there was a disconnect between patient and person, and it is that gap that needed to be bridged.

Let me illustrate what it meant to be reduced to Patient 123432. At one point during my hospital stay, I was placed under cardiology service. After several days of testing, the cardiologist visited me and said I would be taken off that cardiology service. He left the room. A few minutes later the telephone rang and I was holding a conversation when the nurse and an assistant walked in. While I was still talking, they proceeded to reach into my gown to remove the tabs that were there for cardiac monitoring. When they got down to a certain point, they lifted my breast, at which point I stopped and asked them if they would wait until I finished my conversation. They said nothing and walked out. I felt that my personhood had been violated.

On another occasion, when I was hooked up to poles on my right and on my left, unable to move, I rang the call button for assistance in going to the restroom. I waited for what seemed like a lifetime. When someone finally came, the retort was, "You are not the only patient on the floor." Clearly, I could not move unassisted. It was such a demeaning experience I wanted to cry.

When I was discharged from the hospital, I was given the usual discharge paper. I had this pink sheet of paper in my hand but had no idea of its significance. Some days later I read it. I saw

"Colon Adenocarcinoma Stage III." I had no idea what that meant. I thought, "Well, what is Stage III?" As soon as I was able to, I went to a bookstore and found as many books as I could on the subject. I left with two shopping bags full. I read and read.

My recovery and recuperation went as expected. Then came chemotherapy. I said to significant others, "I have never been down this path before. I need someone to walk with me, hold my hand, wipe my tears. Yet, while I was coping with my emotions, I also had a tremendous "need to know."

The weeks of recuperation passed—and then the onset of chemotherapy (Leucovorin and Fluorouracil (5–FU))—from April through December. It was the hardest thing I ever experienced. Going from office to office, lab to lab, clinic to clinic; sitting around for hours and hours, most times in an area that was miserably cold. Most of the time, I was there alone. I prayed audibly, I talked to God audibly, I sang audibly—all this enabled me to keep my sanity and helped to relieve my depression.

I recall, on one of my most difficult days, wanting a glass of water. The chemotherapy had so weakened me that I could not get out of bed and there was no one there to get it for me. It took sheer willpower and determination to finally move from my bedroom to my kitchen. There I got a can of Ensure and a small bottle of water and returned to my bed with both in hand. I knew I had to make it.

That was a turning point in my psychic struggle. I realized that it was God's will that I should live and that I should live abundantly. I knew He would help heal me because there was more on this earth that He had for me to do.

There were passages in scripture that gave me strength; one, in particular, I want to share here from Peter 5:10–11: "After you have suffered a little while, our God, who is full of kindness through Christ, will give you his eternal glory. He personally will come and pick you up, and set you firmly in place, and make you stronger than ever. To Him be all power over all things, forever and ever. Amen." *(The Living Bible Paraphrased)*

There are many blessings that have come from my brokenness. I was given wonderful support from family, friends, pastors, and my congregation. This is a new season of my life. As a consequence of my cancer experience, I have a new mission in life, a new life purpose.

God has used me to start a non-profit organization that focuses on cancer prevention and early detection for persons who are uninsured, underinsured, and medically underserved. It is an awesome vision that He has given me. This is the most wonderful time of my life.

Through God's grace and mercy, I am sharing my journey with others—offering education, financial assistance, encouragement, support, compassion, and comfort.

I learned, and I will share this nugget of wisdom with the reader; that we know our own bodies better than anyone else. If something is wrong, don't stop until you have what you think is a plausible explanation. Most of all, God is in charge of everything. Just as He used my voice to ask for a certain procedure, He will make His presence known to all who call His name. Trust and obey.

GRACE L. BUTLER, PH.D.

CHAPTER EIGHT

Lean on Me

FROM THE SURGERY TO DETERMINE WHETHER OR NOT
THERE WAS A MALIGNANCY THROUGH THE SURGERY
FOR REMOVAL OF THE MALIGNANT TISSUE (A PARTIAL
RADICAL MASTECTOMY) AND THE REMOVAL OF LYMPH
NODES TO DETERMINE WHETHER OR NOT THE CANCER
HAD SPREAD, I SUDDENLY BECAME WHOLLY
DEPENDENT UPON THE KINDNESS OF MY FRIENDS. I
HAD TO DEPEND ON MY FRIENDS FOR MY PERSONAL
CARE, FOR THE WALKING OF MY DOG, FOR THE
SECUREMENT OF GROCERIES, FOR THE COOKING AND
SERVING OF FOOD, FOR THE CLEANING UP OF THE
KITCHEN AND OF THE HOUSE, FOR TRANSPORTATION
TO AND FROM THE DOCTORS, FOR THE HANDLING OF
CORRESPONDENCE, AND FOR DIPLOMATIC DEALING
WITH INNUMERABLE PHONE CALLS: FOR MY LIFE.

—June Jordan

Blanche

What happens when cancer strikes in the twilight of life? How does an almost ninety-year-old women cope with needing to give care to a husband of nearly sixty years?

I am the daughter of a former slave and I am also a former civilian nurse in the U.S. Army. I am eighty-nine years old and take care of my husband, Dr. Thomas Bridge, who is eighty-two. We have been married for fifty-seven years. My husband was the chair of the music department at Virginia State University in Ettrick, Virginia. I graduated from the Freedman's School of Nursing, now the Howard University School of Nursing, in 1938. Tommy's father was a laborer in a Detroit auto factory and his mother was musically inclined. A concert violinist, Dr. Bridge was one of the first African Americans to be selected to play in the Richmond Symphony Orchestra.

Two years ago, Tommy was diagnosed with prostate cancer. Despite regular checkups, his PSA was found to be very high. All of a sudden his PSA went through the roof. It was a shock to say the least. He also had problems walking and had a pain in the hip and we couldn't find out what was causing it. The orthopedic surgeon did a hip replacement and that's when they found out. I think the fact that it was not caught earlier was an oversight. Tommy's illness was a shock to everyone and it completely changed our lives together. Now I have to do everything.

My husband comes from the old school. We don't talk about the cancer much. He just doesn't want to talk about it. The doctors told us that they are taking care of it and so we don't talk about it. We just go on and live our lives.

Tommy thinks he can do more than he can. At a Christmas party, he tried to walk up a slight incline, but he couldn't make it and I couldn't help him. So two strong, younger men had to carry him into the party. He didn't like that much, but he joked, "That's the first time someone has carried me into a party and not out of it!"

His spirit is still very strong. That's why he thinks he can do more than he can do. He thinks he's supposed to do better than anyone else and not give in to things. That's what his generation was brought up to believe.

I cannot handle my husband's condition by myself, especially at night. That's when he often falls down, even when he uses a walker. There's a "young man" (a neighbor over fifty) across the street who helps me pick him up. If Tommy falls down, I call the young man and he comes over to help. We started off with friends staying overnight, but Tommy didn't want anyone sitting up and looking at him in his bedroom. He said he wasn't going to have that. Now I need more help, so I have registered with an in-home hospice care service.

Despite our problems, I'm going to try to hang onto him as long as I can. Sometimes I get a little depressed about it. But we're doing everything we can to keep him mobile and active. Sometimes it's hard because I have to do all of things he used to do—keeping up with the bills, the house, making sure everything gets done. He did so much for fifty years. Sometimes I don't know how he did it.

Tommy has been a good husband to me all of our lives. He's always been a caring, sensitive, and thoughtful husband. I'm grateful for that. If I were in his position, he would do everything for me, so I have to do everything for him.

I don't think about what life would be like without him. I don't have the time and I'm really not at that point yet.

BLANCHE BRIDGE

Christine

Christine is a former registered nurse at King's County Hospital in New York City and a wife and caregiver to a prostate cancer survivor.

My husband has survived for over five years after getting the news that he had prostate cancer. He is one of the three men in my life with the disease. My ex-husband and my brother also have prostate cancer. They all rely on me for comfort and advice. However, only my current husband really looked the disease in the eye and did what he had to do—that is, have surgery.

Some men are afraid of prostate surgery. They think, "I'm not going to let them do this to me." But my husband was a physical education teacher and I was a registered nurse. We knew quite a bit about prostate cancer before this happened, but we learned more from our terrific oncologist, who was very thorough about explaining the options to us. My husband was sixty at the time and we wanted to be sure that the surgeon removed as much of the disease as possible the first time, without having to go back and cut a little more and go back again if that didn't work.

The strange thing about my husband's experience is that he found the disease himself. The doctor had missed it during one of his yearly checkups. But my husband went back about a week later and told the doctor he had detected something. Well, the doctor did more intensive tests and sure enough, my husband had prostate cancer.

When first I heard about it, I got that scared feeling you get when you hear the word "cancer." But I was just glad he found it when he did. Imagine what could have happened at his age if he had missed it. I thank God it was found in time.

To me, it's like my husband had a bad heart attack. He couldn't do certain things, like after a stroke. So I had to pitch in to help. After he recovered, my husband became so active in the American Cancer Society that you'd think that it was his job. They called him to speak about prostate cancer to many groups.

We are okay now and my husband still works for the American Cancer Society, but he has slowed down a bit. After all, he's getting older. But don't tell him I said so.

My brother, too, has prostate cancer. He didn't have surgery. But now his PSA is up and they don't know why. If he had had it removed in the first place, I don't think he would have all of these problems.

I think my brother is just plain stubborn. He's an ex-master sergeant and thinks he is invincible. However, he is coming around a bit. Now, he goes to the VA hospital and carefully follows his PSA. My brother had a lot of discipline. When the doctor told him that he had fluid on his heart, he stopped smoking and drinking the next day and hasn't touched cigarettes or alcohol since.

My ex-husband is another story. He told me that he was going to leave his prostate cancer in God's hands. I told him to go in and have the surgery, but so far he won't listen to either our children or me. He lives in New York City. When I visit there, I have to coax him. "Go to the doctor and see why your PSA is up," I tell him. He will say something like, "Nothing's wrong with me. I'm alright. Whatever is going to happen to me is going to happen to me." I think that he is on a guilt trip that we're no longer together.

The three men in my life who have prostate cancer all come to me with their problems. I talk to them about it. But I stopped talking so much to my ex-husband. I don't think he is going to do anything about it. My daughter, who is forty years old now, moved from Florida to New York to make sure that she is close to her father, but even she can't get him to take good care of himself. I feel that he is punishing himself for what happened in our past. That's not necessary. I say, let the past just be the past.

My husband still loves to talk to groups about prostate cancer. We both think that's important. Our African-American men need not be so afraid when they get the news that they have the disease. And they shouldn't be afraid to learn about it either. They need to remember that the longer they wait, the worse it gets. They should just ask for a PSA when their blood is drawn for other tests during an annual checkup.

I think men like my ex-husband, who want to leave it in God's hands, are making a big mistake. God needs help, too. That's why we have doctors and physical examinations. As far as my ex-husband is concerned, I really believe that had I stayed with him, this would not have happened. He still listened to me, so I would have pushed him to do the right thing.

I'm afraid that the disease may be in his bones now because one of his legs is bent. He never had that before. He says that he will be all right. But I don't believe him. When I'm around he won't walk and he has fallen down a few times. His idea that he will be alright isn't real, especially with this kind of cancer. You do not get to be alright with this disease by ignoring it.

MRS. CHRISTINE SCHOFIELD

Krystal

Krystal's grandmother and her aunt fought their cancers together. Krystal, who was healthy, helped the older women through the hard times and in their times of peril. Krystal grew during the experience. She knows the power of love and she also knows the importance for her, an African-American woman, to take care of her body.

We haven't been formally introduced, but we are all connected through a common bond. I have not had cancer, but I have mentally, emotionally, and socially felt the ramifications of this plight that plagues our community.

The word cancer has been a part of my life for at least twelve years. I do not remember the exact year my grandmother, Esther Lee Wardford, felt that lump in her breast that was later found to be the size of a grapefruit; however, I do remember that it was in March, 2002, that my virtuous aunt, Bevelyn Ann, found that she had ovarian cancer. Who would have known a sharp sensation of pain in her pelvis would send her world in a totally different direction?

I was confused when I came home from college in the summer of 2002 to find that my aunt had lost all her beautiful gray hair. I was confused because although the chemotherapy was designed to make her better, at times it was like poison running through her veins. Now, I wonder when she will get the feeling back in her sometimes lifeless hands and feet. I am happy to see that now she is able to walk without discomfort because for so long she was not able to wear shoes. Family, this statement is not meant to scare you, but I want you to know that cancer treatment can be painful. But remember, each experience is different and some people come through treatment with only a few serious side effects.

My grandmother's experience with chemo was a little disturbing because at one point her doctor gave her an overdose. Our family was concerned that she would not allow us to take legal action against the medical facility. As the years went by, several of my grandmother's friends who had been diagnosed at the same time as she was, passed away. My grandmother believed that maybe she was blessed to live so much longer in spite of that medical mix-up. Still the radiation left her body with third degree burns and lasting scars.

Many people take this journey and there are so many things that can happen. In the end, I know that there is definitely a God who has control over our destiny and, no matter what we think, He is the only pilot of these vessels known as "our bodies."

As I grow in age and in faith I also know it is imperative that as an African-American woman I take care of my body. I want you, family, whether you are male or female, to make sure to stay together as a family, because the strength and love in this unit are the only things that have brought my aunt out of the darkness and into the light. The strength and dedication that my grandmother always exemplified makes me strong enough to bear life's challenges because she never complained. My grandmother has now gone on to Glory.

KRYSTAL L. WARDFORD

Magnolia

Magnolia knows a lot about cancer. Not only has she worked with cancer patients, but several members of her family have succumbed to the disease. From these experiences, she's drawn some important lessons.

I have lost a few family members to cancer and I have also worked with cancer patients as a medical worker. I don't like to say the "C" word or think about it, but we have to face the reality that this disease is very common in the African-American community. Right now I have an aunt who has just been diagnosed with cancer, but she is coping very well. She acts and talks so positively that she has made me a stronger person and given me the strength to deal with the little things I go through in my life. I also think my aunt gets her strength from her religious background and her faith in God.

My aunt is almost 70. Right now she is undergoing treatment and eating a healthy diet. She is still very strong and has her mental health. From her courage I learned not to take anything for granted. Even on a bad day, I try to be positive because I know there is someone out there who might be in worse condition than I am.

If we have faith and are strong, we can deal with anything that comes our way. Now that I have lost a few family members to cancer, I look at life in a different way. I get my annual checkup, the whole works. I try very hard to eat healthy. I walk as often as I can. I surround myself with positive things and people. I pray daily. Sometimes I meditate. I try not to let people get under my skin much. I try to keep a focused mind. I try not to worry much about things, because I cannot fix everything in this world. I give a smile even if I don't get one back, even on a bad day, but at least I try not to complain.

MAGNOLIA RUSSELL

Daryel

Daryel is an inmate. He could only stare at his dark prison cell and imagine what his father and then his mother were going through as they battled cancer. He knew that they faced physical pain and he felt complex emotions of guilt, sorrow and loneliness. Now both parents have passed away and Daryel feels even more alone.

I am part of a voice that oftentimes goes unheard, a voice muffled by other thunderous noises entombed within steel and concrete walls. I am a prisoner. It is in the spirit of my father and mother, Elbert Lee Burnett, Jr., and Ruth Burnett, both cancer victims, that I was inspired to share these words. I am not a cancer survivor, but I hope that my parent's life experiences will inspire people who are free to commit their time and resources to supporting people, especially little children, suffering from this horrible and painful disease. People with cancer, and people in general, should not have to face their fears and uncertainties by themselves. Sometimes it is easy for the human spirit to be overwhelmed by sadness, grief, and loneliness.

When my father was first diagnosed with cancer, it seemed like my small world came to a standstill. Not being there physically during his time of greatest need made my heart feel a thousand times heavier. Being in prison in some ways shields one emotionally from having to experience the day-to-day painful suffering and mental and physical deterioration that people go through on the outside. But being away from loved ones during times of crisis and adversity causes a throbbing ache that never seems to subside. It is a feeling of guilt and of letting loved ones down in their time of need.

Being in prison means being totally dependent on mail for news, since phone calls are allowed only on an emergency basis. During the months that my father received chemo treatment, I got news only now and then and that made my fear and anxiety worse. My mother would write telling me that my father would only have to undergo a certain number of chemo treatments and that the doctors assured her that everything would be all right. My father kept telling me not to worry about him because his life was in God's hands. Sometimes I felt, while reading my mother's letters, that the doctors were giving her a false sense of hope and that she really did not want to deal with the possibility that my father, her soulmate for 50 years, was dying. Life without him would be inconceivable for her.

A few months after the original diagnosis, the cancer had spread throughout his entire body and he was given less than two weeks to live. I was given one phone call and it would be the last time I would hear his voice or my mother's. A week later he passed away. In some ways it was a relief from the many days and nights he spent in excruciating pain.

A couple of weeks after his home-going services, I received a letter saying that my mother had breast cancer. My mother had written to assure me that she was in good health, but in fact she had refused chemotherapy and other medicines. When my father passed away, a part of her spirit died. I suggested to my sister that she encourage our mother to join a women's support group, which might have helped her deal with her grief and enormous sense of loss in a better way. My sister said my mother never recovered from the loss of my father. I had stopped hearing from my mother; it was like she didn't want to be a burden. A mother can never be a burden. I felt so guilty that I was not available to comfort or to hold the one woman who had given me her love unconditionally. I felt so useless as a son, a brother, and a man.

A year after my father passed away, my mother died of breast cancer. My sister said there was a 90 percent chance of my mother surviving this cancer, but she didn't want to experience, or put other family members through her suffering. She quietly lost her will and purpose to live. I thank God for the strength of my family, especially my sister's and nieces' resiliency. They held things together for us all. The final time my sister kissed my mother she told her that I loved her and my mother said, "I know."

This is my story, in honor and in memory of my parents' and sister Denise Burnett, who died suddenly after a life-long battle against lupus.

Daryel Burnett

Walter

Walter loved his aunts but he was unable to be with them during their dying days or to go to their funerals. Walter is an inmate of Louisiana State Prison. When his mother became ill with breast cancer, Walter was able to research programs that would help her. Still, the prison walls close tighter on him as he wrestles with his guilt and remorse.

Hello, my name is Walter Anthony Johnson and I am a thirty-two-year-old African American currently confined at the Louisiana State Prison in Angola. I'm writing you to share some of my past experiences of how cancer affected my life and my loved ones' lives. I write this letter with all due sincerity and I hope that your readers don't view me in a negative stereotypical light because I'm confined.

I was born and raised in New Orleans, Louisiana. I have three sisters and a beautiful, strong-willed mother named Rose Marie Johnson. My biological father was never there for me. During my upbringing, my mother and two of my aunts, Alice Garrison and

Helen Cline, played some very caring and loving roles in my life. During my confinement, both have passed away from different forms of cancer and the pain has been unbearable. Not to mention my mother, who was recently diagnosed with breast cancer.

At first my mother tried to conceal her illness from me. In a way she was right but what hurts me most is that I am not sure if she is getting the kind of family support she needs.

I was very close to both of my aunts when they passed, yet I was not allowed to go to the funerals. These experiences, along with other chapters in my life compelled me to learn more about different forms of cancer and how cancer affects people's lives.

From prison I tried my best to inform my mother about the few government programs set up to offer help to poor, breast cancer patients in Louisiana. One in particular is the program ENCOREplus in Baton Rouge. After thorough research, I found that they are devoted to helping underprivileged, lower-income African Americans. My mother was able to get some help from them. I've even started learning about mammograms, chemotherapy, and radiation treatment.

I received many letters from my aunts before they passed away, but I was powerless to help them. In my mind, body, and soul, I would give my life to stop the suffering of my mother. Yet, as you should well know, our fates are inevitable.

I also have a few friends confined with me whose mothers endured what my mother is enduring. So, never for one moment from this day forth should you feel alone. Wherever you are, there are always people in this world that care.

WALTER ANTHONY JOHNSON

Deborah

By accident, Deborah stopped by her uncle's house, and found him paralyzed on one side and able to speak only with a slur. For two months she took time off from her job to be with her uncle in the hospital every day. She thinks of her relationship with her uncle as "a big gift." Giving to someone else has deepened her life and strengthened her.

Last December, while moving furnishings from my office, I stopped by my uncle's house to drop off a cabinet. I found him in a state where he seemed like a stroke victim. His speech was slurred and one side of his body was somewhat stiff.

I contacted my mom (his sister), and we took him to a Veterans Hospital. Tests showed evidence of two tumors one on his lung and one on his brain. My uncle was a smoker since he'd served in the Navy during the Korean War. However, he was never sick during his adult life. Other than an appendectomy at seven, he was never in a hospital for anything until I found him stricken at 73, with cancer. I became the primary caregiver and almost a member of the hospital team.

Some folks thought I was a new staff member because I was on board so much. I needed to make sure that he ate and cooperated with the staff. He had spent a lifetime as a lone ranger, doing things his own way. Following the hospital routines was challenging for him, but I did what I could to encourage him. People often commented that I must be his daughter because I was so devoted.

He had no wife and no children. He had mom and me. He was ours. Working with him, I had two purposes: 1) that he realize how much he was loved and 2) that my mom be spared undue stress.

Each morning I went to his bedside. I went to therapy with him and joined in helping him with it as much as I could. He had brain surgery the Tuesday after Christmas 2002. He came through like a champ—a real Navy guy. But following the surgery it seems as if he decided to "opt" out of the whole matter. He shut himself down by refusing to eat and drink fluids. He felt that it was time. God called him home on February 8, 2003. He was saved from further agony. I had prepared to stay off work for the ten months doctors said he had left. The big gift was to be with him each day.

The great irony was that in the past I had always gone in and out, visiting him for only moments. During this strange, unusual time, I was glad to be with him for hours on end. I'd like to be there today with him relaxing and looking at TV. My heart is broken by this. Yet God made the human heart to withstand heavy loads. It heals itself in time.

DEBORAH JACKSON

CHAPTER NINE

Each One Teach One

OUR LABOR HAS BECOME
MORE IMPORTANT
THAN OUR SILENCE.

—Audre Lord, *The Black Unicorn*

Zora

Zora is a well-known breast cancer activist. She founded both the Breast Cancer Resource Committee, (an educational organization) and Rise Sister Rise, a support group for African-American women. Zora's three-decade experience with breast cancer is just one part of her personal journey. Many women in her family have survived the disease, and many have succumbed. Zora's calling is to educate society, emphasizing the value of hope in cancer recovery and survival. She has also continued her personal growth during her long experience with breast cancer.

Although I am a twenty-two-year breast cancer survivor, breast cancer was a journey that began before I was born. Both my grandmother and great-grandmother had breast cancer at a time when little was known of this disease and there was very little reason for hope. Mammography had not yet been invented; genetic factors were unknown; radical mastectomy was virtually the only treatment option, and the survival statistics were grim. People knew so little about breast cancer that they discussed it in whispers—a secret shame. They disguised mention of cancer with euphemisms, calling it the big "C" or "Woman's Disease" or just "IT." So powerful was the stigma in previous generations that women kept silent about it.

A generation later, my mother, also challenged with breast cancer, would face some of the same limitations. Nevertheless, she found the strength to cast off the chains of shame, embarrassment, and perceived personal failure to use her knowledge of family history and emerging medical advances to forge a way toward truth and light. So unfettered was my mother by shame and misconceptions that she was able to pass along to her offspring a sense of knowledge, optimism, and hope.

My mother's faith translated into a glimmer of hope that made my own personal journey dramatically different from my grandmother's and great-grandmother's. The hope of their generation of breast cancer patients, who suffered through the silent stigma of this dreaded disease, transformed into action my mother's desire for better chances of recovery. Indeed, such sustained hopes spawned medical miracles like mammography and gave rise to advances in surgical techniques, genetic screening, chemotherapy, and hormonal therapy. All of these developments have enabled us to watch for signs of cancer, to detect it earlier, to treat tumors before they spread, and even, as previous generations could not, to contemplate an ultimate cure for cancer.

Hope operates on both a personal and collective level in recovery and survival. Personally, hope enables cancer patients to find the will and strength to fight for life in the face of devastating diseases like breast, lung, colon, and pancreatic cancers. Hope is about holding your head high in the face of a silent enemy. Hope encourages you to incorporate tools beyond medicine—such as humor, spirituality and a positive outlook—to fight cancer. Hope enables cancer patients to strive toward insurmountable victories each and every day. It keeps us striving not only towards recovery but also, in many instances, to rebounding and becoming stronger and better than before. From the breast cancer patient regaining enough strength to raise her arm over her head to the lung cancer patient being able to compete in marathons, hope transforms patients from victims into victors.

Hope is the internal whisper that encourages us to keep going for chemotherapy, despite the nausea and hair loss; it makes us show up for radiation treatments, despite dry mouth or skin pigmentation. Occasionally hope shouts at us, encouraging victory to all cancer patients one day at a time, until we are one week, five years or, like myself, twenty-two years down the road of recovery. It's about transforming fear into knowledge: knowledge about family history, medical advances, and strategies for fighting cancer which are all borne out of hope. A better understanding of one's personal history, one's risk for getting the disease, and one's options after being diagnosed with the disease, all lead to the likelihood of satisfying the prevailing hope of all cancer patients—beating the disease.

Hope resonates in a social context because cancer impacts so many lives, either directly or indirectly. Physicians, researchers, therapists, politicians, authors, singers, and painters, whether directly affected or not, utilize hope just like patients, as the impetus for action, breeding new developments that bring us all closer to victory over the disease. Hope exists in all spheres and strata of the social milieu, from corporate boardrooms to legislative chambers. In these realms, hope manifests itself in a call to action, changes in budgets, recognition of corporate responsibility, and an image or song that inspires us to continue our progress on the road to recovery. This collective hope results in a positive cycle that generates more hope: as patients hope, they inspire doctors, who inspire researchers, who inspire others to maintain their hope and continue working on new legislation, new research, new medicines, new therapies, and other advances that make recovery easier and a cure for cancer a real possibility. Because we have hope, my generation doesn't have to resign itself to inevitable death.

Overall, hope is as essential to cancer recovery and survival as medical treatment. In many instances, treatment for cancer is nearly as debilitating as the disease itself. Hope enables the cancer patient to continue, despite the illness, despite the seemingly insurmountable path to recovery, through remission until the day there is a cure.

Hope has enabled me to walk this path of life—each day making me more hopeful that my fellow sisters and brothers— will smell the sweet smell of hope.

ZORA KRAMER BROWN

Ronald

Ronald and Calvin formed the Brother-to-Brother Support Group from their own experiences of isolation and lack of information for African-American men concerning prostate cancer. The group, affiliated with the

American Cancer Society, helps African-American men and their partners cope with this disease.

I was diagnosed with cancer in June 1988. I considered surgery until my doctors decided that external beam radiation would be the best possible treatment since I had had a major heart attack before. The course of treatment recommended by my doctor was the best course of action. I have now been in remission for more than five years.

Recognizing the need of cancer education in the African-American community, I co-founded The Brother-to-Brother Group in June of 1988 with Calvin Martin. Both Calvin Martin and I discovered, after his prostate cancer diagnosis, that there was no place for African-American and Latino men to go for support and information about a disease that affects more African-American and Latino men that other cancers combined. We then decided that something had to be done.

The Brother-to-Brother support program is specially designed for men who have prostate cancer. The purpose of the program is to provide accurate information about diagnosis, treatment options, living with the effects of treatment and other related issues. Men and their partners are able to ask questions, share common experiences, get the assistance of qualified health professionals, and find comfort through the camaraderie of the group. This program also promotes awareness of prostate cancer as a major health concern for men. Men and their partners can greatly benefit from the program and that participation can begin immediately following diagnosis. This is especially important to help reduce anxiety and facilitate a healthy adjustment to the disease.

RONALD BAKER

William

William didn't just take charge of his own prostate cancer treatment. He went further by becoming an advocate for awareness in the Washington D.C. area and in Virginia, which has an extremely high rate of prostate cancer in African-American men. He currently works with the Virginia Prostate Cancer Coalition.

My nine-month checkup after proton treatment reflects a PSA of 1.14, down from the initial PSA of 3.56. For me, this marks a very bright moment that follows a long ordeal.

My journey started with a routine examination by my primary physician in June, 2001, and it ended after 40 radiation treatments at the Loma Linda Proton Center in September, 2002. I went through the treatment that reduced the PSA count without any noticeable side effects.

My wife and I had lived for three years in northern Virginia, near Washington, D.C., after moving there from Redlands, California. So I was interested to read in the paper that a new proton technology was being installed at Loma Linda University Cancer Institute in California. "That's amazing," I said. "Thank God I'll never have to use that." So much for my prophetic powers. Twelve and a half years later I reported to the Proton Unit for treatment.

I had my first indication that something might be wrong during my annual examination in June, 2001. My primary physician, after performing the hated digital rectal exam (DRE), made this offhand comment: "Something doesn't feel quite right. I'm sending you to Walter Reed [I'm in the military medical system] to see a urologist." My PSA was in the 'normal' range, less than four, but there was an area on my prostate that didn't feel right. My primary physician wanted somebody to take a closer look and perhaps do a biopsy.

The urologist at Walter Reed said that he understood why the primary care physician scheduled a visit. Something definitely did not feel right. He asked that I come back in a week for a biopsy. The first, second, and third biopsies were all inconclusive. The part of my anatomy where all of the poking and probing was taking place is sacrosanct to all of us macho-type individuals. That said, imagine the kind of willpower that I had to muster to place myself in the hands of people performing a biopsy for a fourth time.

I frankly did not think that anything was awry with my health because I felt very healthy. Even though I lost my father to prostate cancer in 1989, I believed that a PSA in the "normal" range, below four, coupled with the inconclusive biopsy results, made all of those shenanigans a waste of time.

A few days after my fourth biopsy, the fateful call came from my urologist telling me, "You have prostate cancer with a Gleason score of 7." I had no idea what a Gleason score was, but I did know I had cancer and that my wife and I should take a logical approach to this challenge. My urologist, during the same conversation made an appointment for me to see him the following week for a consultation and to go over my treatment choices.

The evening that I received that dreaded call, my wife, bless her heart, went directly to the Internet and started the research process. We both knew that prostate cancer was slow moving but we wanted to look at all the options and be prepared prior to our visit with the urologist. We came to the conclusion, after much investigation, that Loma Linda and its Proton Program was the best option for suppressing the disease and letting me maintain a good quality of life.

When I met with the urologist, I had already decided what path I was going to take, but I listened to his "sales pitch." According to him, I had only two choices, surgery or radiation. He gave me a laundry list of side effects and potential problems that could occur from both surgery and radiation and also recommended that I visit the radiation unit for consultation. He told me that if I chose surgery, I should let him know by no later than the following week so that he could work it into his schedule.

What the urologist didn't know was that Loma Linda had already accepted me into the program. I asked him about proton treatment at Loma Linda. He told me that Walter Reed had sent a couple of people there for treatment and, as far as he knew, it was good treatment. We agreed that I had to begin on this program within five months.

I had another hurdle to negotiate before getting into the Loma Linda program. The upper weight limit was 255 pounds, because treatment requires the patient to fit properly into the "half casket" or pod. I was 320 pounds in January, but the five-month waiting window afforded me the opportunity to trim myself down. I started eating healthy, 1800 calories a day, and did strength training and cardio for two-to-three hours, six days a week. By July 2nd, I had successfully lost the weight, coming in at three pounds under the limit.

Cancer gave me a positive platform for change that I still maintain: I have lost another 35 pounds on my way to my goal of 200 pounds, a goal I will reach by late summer, 2003. A welcome side effect of this weight loss is that I was able to get off my diabetes medication. It seems as if diet, exercise, and weight loss do, in fact, go a long way toward diabetes control.

I was accepted into the Proton Program in February, 2002, and scheduled to report on July 1, 2002. The good news was that we were going home! Children, grandchildren, and relatives would be happy distractions. In fact, once I arrived at Loma Linda, the main challenge was keeping focused.

I soon realized how blessed I was to be a part of such a program. At my first Wednesday support group, I heard a talk by a "graduate" named Alex Plummer. I was very impressed with his efforts to give something back to the African-American high-risk community. I drove to Pasadena to talk further with Alex and I left armed with telephone numbers and ideas for pursuing efforts like his in the Washington/Baltimore area.

I gleaned some very scary statistics from an article written by Courtland Milloy in the January 29, 2003, edition of the *Washington Post*. African-American men in the nation's capital have one of the highest rates of prostate cancer in the world; in fact, according to the American Cancer Society, 600 cases of prostate cancer will be diagnosed each year and of those 600 cases, 100 will die.

Such deaths can be counted in advance, year after year. Why? Michael Richardson, interim chief medical officer for the D. C. Department of Health, said, "We know people won't see a doctor unless they are bleeding from some orifice, by then it may be too late." CeCe Dorough, programs manager for the National Prostate Cancer Coalition said that many African-American men don't understand the disease and "may not feel comfortable talking about prostate cancer because it occurs in a part of the body that represents their manhood." For those who believe manhood emanates from between their legs, a mental makeover is prescribed. Maybe that would help some men put mind over matter when it comes to those intrusive exams.

Theories abound about why African Americans have such a high rate of prostate cancer. These theories range from diet to genetics. Michael J. Manyak, chairman of the Department of

Urology at George Washington University, stated, "The wild card in all of this is genetics. There is research on whether Black and White men metabolize testosterone differently and in such a way that accelerates growth of prostate cancer in Black men." Doctors say that the proper response is for African-American men to become more vigilant and begin screening for prostate cancer by age forty, instead of by age fifty as is recommended for White men.

Those without adequate health coverage are automatically placed at a disadvantage. I hope that someday we will change that but for the time being, if free screening is not available the average cost of a prostate exam is $70. A follow-up biopsy is approximately $1500 and, if cancer is detected, conventional treatment alone can cost as much as $30,000.

I am currently on the speakers bureau with the Virginia Prostate Cancer Coalition and I am on a mission to talk to as many Black organizations as I can to promote awareness. I am also working with Dr. David Bostwick of the Bostwick Laboratories in Richmond to develop a comprehensive medical repository for cancer patients. This program, should it be implemented, will allow physicians to recommend the type of treatment needed based upon the particular diagnosis of the patient.

This journey has been incredible on many levels. I have met so many wonderful, supportive people and I am keeping in touch with other cancer survivors that I have met through the support functions.

I appreciate the opportunity to share my story in the hope that it will benefit others. I am looking forward to a long, fruitful relationship with all of the support groups that I am affiliated with and invite conversation through e-mail or telephone if anyone has any questions or comments.

WILLIAM D. JACKSON

Mike

Mike was prepared to die after he was diagnosed with prostate cancer. Five years later, he is cancer-free and an advocate for prostate health for African Americans in Sacramento.

I was a 48-year-old African-American man, retired from the military. Having just completed the requirements for my bachelors degree and being in pretty decent health, I was ready to tackle "corporate America." I applied for and was accepted for a position with a now defunct company in California.

I went for a physical exam, after which my doctor informed me that something "felt suspicious." He asked me questions about symptoms but I did not have any symptoms that would have indicated an illness. After undergoing other exams, I received a call from my doctor who tried to sensitize his tone but "you have cancer" cannot be soft-shoed. I believed that there must be a mistake, so my doctor agreed to see me the next day without an appointment. He showed me X-rays and lab reports. I was looking at my prostate but I couldn't admit to myself or my wife that I had cancer.

After returning home, I couldn't hide the look on my face from my wife. We sat alone and I told her. The thought of being dead at 48, with my wife left to raise our newly adopted grandchildren was unbearable. At that time, in my mind those were real thoughts. After 40 or so minutes of crying and praying we regrouped. I updated my will, called my mom and sister in Chicago, and found the courage to tell them of my impending death. I had accepted what I thought was my fate and was honestly prepared to die.

The next day, my doctor called and asked me to bring my wife with me for a visit. At the visit, I was given videotapes of other Black men who also had survived prostate cancer. My wife and I watched a couple of tapes and afterwards, it hit me. This is not the 'death sentence' I envisioned. This time my tears were tears of joy. I said my blessings and "Thank you" to my Lord and Savior.

My doctor discussed various treatments with my wife and me. After agreeing to surgery to remove my prostate, I never looked back. The thought of death was indeed a self-imposed scare tactic.

It has now been five years and counting. I'm still cancer free. I've been a self-proclaimed "poster boy" for the African-American Prostate Cancer Support Group here in Sacramento. What I think is key to dealing with and surviving prostate cancer is awareness and education. We must continue to spread the word and help people relieve doubts. If I knew then what I know now about prostate cancer, death would not have occupied my mind. Simple as that!

It is sad but true that many men would prefer "not to know" and some will never allow a male doctor to perform the necessary examinations. "It's a dirty job but somebody gets paid to do it." I want to know about my body and if I have to pay somebody to tell me, so be it!

I have a large family and I traced my genealogy back to my great-grandparents on my mom's and dad's sides. There was never a case of any kind of cancer. I am the eldest of ten siblings. At my urging and nagging, my four brothers and my cousin have had exams and all are clean. All of them are over 40. Now I'm telling them about colonoscopies!

Thank you for taking the time to read this.

MIKE TRUMAN

Ola

Ola Mae said she "always had lumpy breasts," but never went in for an examination. After an exam, her doctor discovered that she had breast cancer. Chemotherapy, which she calls "the best birthday present that I've ever had," successfully treated her disease and she has become an advocate for healthy breast care. Ola Mae also remembers her friends that have passed from breast cancer.

In March of 1994, I went for a regular physical examination. During my examination, a lump was found in my right breast. My doctor then referred me to a specialist for a biopsy. The biopsy revealed aggressive breast cancer but, because it was found in an early stage, I was given the option of a mastectomy or a lumpectomy.

My diagnosis was a shock because I had always had lumpy breasts but I never thought I would have breast cancer. At first, I felt like I was having a bad dream; after that I got real depressed. But eventually I began to draw on my spiritual resources and worked to gain all the information I could through books and pamphlets given to me by the American Cancer Society.

On April 21, 1994, I had a lumpectomy. Cancer had spread to two of my lymph nodes, out of the thirty-seven that were taken from my armpit. My doctor recommended that I have radiation and chemotherapy. At the time, I was preparing for two college graduations—my son's graduation from Purdue University in Indiana and my younger daughter's graduation from Cal Poly Pomona in California—so my doctor started me on radiation right away, but put off the chemotherapy until I returned from Indiana.

In July of 1994 I started chemotherapy which I finished on my birthday on December 2nd. Completing chemotherapy was the best birthday present I've ever received.

I had little support, only a few contacts that were given to me by the American Cancer Society. Since my challenge, it has made me more sensitive to illness and I feel a greater appreciation for life itself. I have given support to six cancer patients. Three are deceased because of the stage when their cancer was detected. Two are survivors and one is still battling the disease. As a result of my continued healing, I have experienced the birth of two grandchildren and another one will be born soon. I am so grateful to God for my continued healing.

Although this was a very traumatic time in my life, I give all the glory to my Lord and Savior Jesus Christ. He was with me through all of my battles and is still with me today. I thank God for my wonderful husband, Uleses, who was there when I needed his shoulders to cry on and to pray for me, assuring me of his love. I'm also blessed to have my wonderful church family, Faith Center Ministries in Walnut, California, and my doctor, J. Frank Yamanishi, at Kaiser Permanente Hospital in Fontana.

I have been in remission for nine and a half years.

Discovery of a lump in the breast does not always mean that cancer is present. But it does always mean that you should contact your doctor without delay. Ignorance and delay account for many deaths from breast cancer that would not have happened if a small suspicious lump had been called immediately to a physician's attention. When the malignant tumor is localized, then chances of success by surgical removal are excellent.

Remembering my friends that are deceased:
Ms. Etta Parr
Mrs. Mattie Willis
Ms. Shirl McEewn
Mrs. Charlene Jamerson
Mrs. Naomi Smalley

Remembering my friends that are survivors of breast cancer:
Mrs. Carolyn Smith
Ms. Diana Levy
Mrs. Shirley Newton

OLA MAE

Franklin

Franklin was fastidious about getting checkups for prostate cancer and to ensure that he was healthy in general. He had been getting PSA and DREs for nearly a decade. But one year, he had a "suspicion" and prodded his doctors to give him a biopsy. When the results came in, he immediately had surgery and he has been well ever since. In fact, Franklin became the "poster boy" for prostate cancer prevention in Colorado. His message is early detection, education, spiritual strength, and a positive mental outlook.

Most of my life, I've given some thought to how I would react if faced with the dreaded disease of cancer. Although I never dwelled extensively on the thought, it often appeared and I continually pushed such thoughts aside. With little or no effort, I placated myself with thoughts like "Nothing as dreadful as cancer could happen to me. Not to Franklin Clay!" Cancer was the other person's disease and I was not that person. Why should I be concerned? I was fine, just fine!

At age fifty-two, I noticed a slight decrease in my urine flow and I had difficulties in starting and stopping that flow. I knew little about urination problems except what I heard from my peers; and in hindsight, they were not qualified for such medical judgments. My problems were simple; at least that was my thought as I diagnosed myself. I concluded that my problems were natural among all males over the age of fifty, so what was the big deal?

As I became more aware of prostate disease in men, especially in the African-American community, I decided to seek the opinion of a well-qualified urologist. Following an exam with a scope and a digital rectal exam (DRE), I was informed that my prostate was indeed enlarged. However there were no indications of cancer or need for treatment at that time. I was elated and listened intently to the urologist's every word. His instructions were that I continue to be watchful and visit my urologist at least annually, or more often, if I experienced problems in that area.

During the next eight years, I visited my urologist religiously, at least once a year; and I followed his instructions. In November, 1995, small nodules were detected during a routine DRE. My PSA count never elevated above two. Normally an elevation of four or more warrants additional checks. Based on my PSA results, everything looked great regarding my prostate. Because the PSA and DRE must be taken and considered together, my urologist recommended a six-month waiting period to ascertain if any changes occurred in either my DRE or PSA.

Six months later, no major changes were noted, but the element of suspicion was ever present. My urologist and I agreed that it was better to be safe than sorry and we made preparations for additional checks. A sonogram (ultrasound) and a biopsy revealed two cancerous areas. All guessing games were now over. That dreaded thought had become the dreaded reality. I had cancer.

To my amazement, I did not panic. My world did not come to an abrupt end. At age sixty-one, I took stock of my life and found myself looking with great expectation to a long and productive future. Two powerful forces propelled my positive outlook: God Almighty and early detection. Everything was on my side; and if not, I had done my job.

I immediately educated myself about prostate cancer and the different treatment options and I discussed the alternatives with my doctor. My urologist and I agreed that a radical prostatectomy operation would probably offer me the best chance of living longer. It was important that we be equal partners in this decision. In September, 1996, my operation was performed at Evans Army Community Hospital, in Fort Carson, Colorado. God Almighty had conveniently placed all the right people in all the right places. My post operation recovery was a breeze; I was out of the hospital in less than three days and never took a pain pill. The operation was a total success and all possible side effects were nonexistent or very negligible.

For the past seven years, I have passed all my checkups with flying colors. My PSA is at zero, I feel great and the world is a beautiful place. I'm happy with my doctor, but I'm even happier with what I did. I went for regular checkups and I became very aware of my body. I got involved with my healthcare and by the Grace of God, I saved my life.

I have dedicated my life over the past seven years, to spreading the word and educating males, especially African-American males, on the importance of early detection in the management of prostate cancer. I receive so much joy from spreading the word about prostate cancer because I truly believe that I am making a difference and that countless lives are being prolonged because of my commitment and the commitment of others to the cause.

Although I am not as active as I was in the past, I remain supportive. I was instrumental in establishing a chapter of US TOO, a support group for prostate cancer survivors at Fort Carson. I have served as the vice-chairman of the local American Cancer Society's prostate cancer task force and was the 1998 volunteer of the year for the El Paso/Teller County unit of the American Cancer Society. I have appeared on local radio and television and led several successful fundraisers in the fight against cancer. I stand forever ready to answer the call.

Giving thanks to God Almighty who is the sustainer of all life, I would like to close by saying that I helped myself through my ordeal by being aware of good health practices. I have always been an active person. I went into my operation without any conditions like high blood pressure, diabetes, obesity or alcohol problems, problems that are shared by too many African Americans. My doctor was very pleased with my general health.

I encourage all individuals, especially African Americans, to get involved in living a healthier lifestyle. There is something to that old saying that our parents told us in years long gone: "An ounce of prevention is worth a pound of cure."

FRANKLIN CLAY

Denise

Denise Roberts had two young children when she was diagnosed. Today she is a 17 year breast cancer survivor!

In 1987, I was going about my regular routine of living when I noticed that my hair was coming out a little more than usual when I combed it every day. I had also become aware of darkness under my eyes. Some of my close friends made comments about the changes and asked if I was breaking under the pressure. I was 34 with two children, fourteen months apart—my son was seven and my daughter was five. Of course, the last thing on my mind was cancer, but I was concerned about what was happening to me and I wanted an immediate solution.

I had a good OB/GYN and we were always able to communicate well, so I went to him with my strong feeling that there was something wrong with me. He asked all the usual questions and I answered with a new request, I wanted a mammogram. Well, he looked at me with shock and quickly said, "No!" He then explained his answer. First of all, I was 34 years old, I had regular breast exams with my Pap test, and most important, I didn't smoke or drink and I had breast fed both of my children. Also, let's not leave out the 34A breast size! What was I thinking? Well, even with all those so-called wonderful statistics going for me, I still couldn't shake the strong feeling that there was something wrong.

After all the hesitations, I was scheduled for the mammogram. The next day my doctor called and said the mammogram had showed a little "something," so I met with the radiologist who explained he was going to do a needle biopsy. He gave me a shot to numb the right breast and then proceeded to insert a needle into the area where they had seen the "something." I waited for the results with my mother and my sister Jackie, in the hospital lounge. The wait seemed forever, but the news was great! The doctor said the test revealed a benign tumor in my milk duct. I was free to go! I had gotten my satisfaction and there was nothing wrong!

About ten days later, my husband came home and said to me that we needed to see my OB/GYN in the morning. I asked him why, was there something wrong? I looked into his eyes and before he could answer, I knew the truth. Something was definitely wrong with me. He looked so sad and finally said, "You have breast cancer. . . ." His voice was soft and compassionate, but for me it came out strong and loud. It felt like I was having an out-of body experience. I was devastated! How could this happen? Were the doctors lying? I didn't really know how to handle this news. I got up from the side of the bed and just stared at the floor. It was as if I were waiting for my husband to wake me up from this nightmare. After we both stopped crying, I fell asleep and woke up to the realization that there was a possibility that I could die. My husband and I went into my OB/GYN's office and sat before him with heavy hearts.

I had a 1.5 centimeter carcinoma. But I wanted to live! So I went home to prepare myself and my family for surgery. I was set to have a mastectomy two weeks later. When the doctor removed the breast, he found seven more malignant carcinomas in the breast tissue, which he successfully removed. Also, 15 lymph nodes were removed and none had been affected. My whole world was coming apart. I was 35 years old, and had just one boob! I didn't have immediate reconstructive surgery because I was so messed up after having a radical mastectomy. I just wanted to go home and comprehend what was really taking place in my life!

My surgeon had explained that the statistics on women of color getting breast cancer between the ages of 20 and 35 were very high. This was hard for me to believe. I wanted to hear from other African-American women my age about their successful treatments, so he gave me the names of African-American support groups to contact. I was surprised to see how many there were, considering I had never seen any ads or TV coverage with women of color associated with breast cancer. I had only seen or heard about support groups for White women. I went to the support group Women of Color and I was happy to see myself mirrored in these women who had gone through what I thought was the end of the road. I did not feel I could go on with my life in the way I had before I was diagnosed with cancer.

After ten years of living free of breast cancer, I was ready for reconstruction. I was also excited by statistics that showed if there were no signs of cancer after ten years, there was a ninety percent chance of living with no recurrence. I was really ready to put the prosthesis away! I went for my appointment with one of the most renowned reconstructive plastic surgeons on the West Coast. Although I had my scar to remind me that I was still in the war against breast cancer, I was winning!

In 1997, as a successful interior decorator with a design shop, I found myself constantly coming into contact with people who had questions about breast cancer and mammograms. After I gave them advice and supportive answers, they always asked me how I knew just the right answers. When I would tell them that I was a survivor of breast cancer, they looked at me with such disbelief that I just smiled, and gave them strong hugs. That is when I realized that I needed those hugs, and I decided to go after them. I closed my store, retired from decorating and asked my nephew, who is an attorney to help me establish a non-profit organization. I wanted to share with my sisters and brothers the true way of living after being diagnosed with the dreaded disease of breast cancer. After months of working and bringing in more friends to help with the mission statement, I was able to establish the Denise Roberts Breast Cancer Foundation—Minority Women Fighting Breast Cancer. We have been in this war for five years, and I have grown stronger than I ever felt I could.

Every time I give support to a sister by getting her a mammogram or by giving support to the family that has been left behind after the loved one has passed on, I realize that no matter what, we shall keep that commitment to fight for a cure in our lifetime!

DENISE ROBERTS

CODA

The narratives in this book reflect the burgeoning movement within the African-American community to end the silence of cancer. Our voices challenge others to acknowledge our shared histories, as we defy the tradition of secrecy that has engulfed this disease. Our stories were written primarily to validate our own experiences, but more importantly they were shared to educate others about the importance of prevention, early detection, treatment and self-advocacy.

Cancer is not just a disease; it is a revealing journey during which a human reflects on life's pleasures, its pain and its vicissitudes. It is a journey that demands physical, emotional and psychological endurance. And, not the least, it demands time. Before cancer, our time was wholly preoccupied with working, running errands, going to meetings or meeting other set deadlines. But in a flash, our precious time was usurped by treatments, visits to medical professionals or talking to insurance company representatives.

But cancer can also be very giving. It gives us back time, time that we use to connect with our families and friends. We also make time to serve as human resources for our community. So many of us have found ways, even in illness, to become advocates for African-American survival. As advocates we challenge medical practitioners and institutions for equal care; we challenge insurance companies to pay their fair share for our treatment; we challenge pharmaceuticals to consider our special needs in conducting research and in implementing clinical trials; and we challenge corporations and the government to clean the environment.

Yes, cancer is giving. Cancer gives us the wisdom to release pain, anger and regrets. It gives us the vision to see where others are blind. We are more open to love, even loving our enemies. Our cancer experience has released us from concentrating on negativity or simple pettiness. We, more that most people, understand that negative energy serves no useful purpose on our journey. Cancer also reinforces our faith, our faith in a higher power and faith in our ability to use that power for greater purpose.

We applaud our family and friends who stood by us during our journey. We forgive those who could not support us adequately out of fear, anger, or guilt. We appreciate our physicians, nurses, social workers and other professionals who acknowledged our humanity as we endured surgery, radiation and various chemotherapies and alternative treatments. And, we affirm and support the unique journey of others who have been touched by cancer.

Even after all the years spent working on this book, I still marvel at the fact that I was blessed with piloting such a worthy endeavor. The survivors entrusted me to tell their stories and share their message of hope, faith and survival. I hope that I have served them well.

KARIN L. STANFORD

THE DEFEAT WILL NOT BE OURS

WHO ARE YOU, THAT SNEAKS INTO OUR BODIES
LURKING DEEP, TAKING US CELL BY CELL
THROUGH THE REMINDER THAT MORTALITY
AND THE CRUEL VINEGAR OF PAIN
CARE NOTHING FOR TALENT, FOR HOPE, FOR THE PROMISE OF
   SPIRIT

WHAT GIVES YOU THE RIGHT TO STEAL OUR TREASURE?
DON'T YOU SEE OUR PRIDE?
DON'T YOU UNDERSTAND THAT WE HAVE CHILDREN, FAMILY AND
   FRIENDS

YOUR CREDITS ARE IMPRESSIVE
THE LIST NEEDLESSLY LONG
EACH SOUL YOU STOP,
A HERO LOST

AUDRE LORDE, GREGORY HINES, WALTER PAYTON, JOHNNIE
   COCHRAN
BOB MARLEY, HATTIE MCDANIEL, NINA SIMONE, TOO.
THE PIONEERS, LEGENDS WE LOVED
GONE TOO SOON.

YES, WE HOLD HOPE FOR THE ONES THAT BY FORCE OF MIRACLE
ESCAPED YOUR GRASP
GREW STRONGER AND THROVE
COLIN POWELL, DIAHANN CARROLL, ERIC DAVIS
DARRYL STRAWBERRY, RICHARD ROUNDTREE

THE VICTORIES ARE SWEET, BUT CAN'T OUTDO THE BITTER
   SADNESS
OF OUR LOSSES CLOSE AND FAR

WE DON'T WANT TO BE VICTIMS, SURVIVORS, CARETAKERS AND
   THOSE LEFT BEHIND.
NOT YOUR KIND.
ANYMORE.
THE BLESSING OF LIFE IS SHORT ENOUGH WITHOUT YOU
AS OUR MOTHERS, COUSINS, LOVERS AND OTHERS
SLAP AT YOUR GREEDY HANDS, BEG AT YOUR FEET
IF NOT FOR A CURE, THEN FOR AN ANSWER WHY.

EVERY NIGHT WE CLOSE OUR EYES
NOT KNOWING IF THE OTHER SIDE WILL BRING
ANOTHER NEWS REPORT
ANOTHER PHONE CALL
ANOTHER LORRAINE HANSBERRY, JUNE JORDAN, MINNIE
   RIPERTON . . .
ANOTHER SISTER, UNCLE, SON, FRIEND OF OURS . . .

YOURS.

BUT THE DEFEAT WILL NOT BE OURS.

WE GREET EACH DAY WITH THE STRENGTH, WILL AND PRAYERS
THANKFUL, KEEP US
DETERMINED TO FIGHT
TO WIN
NOT JUST SURVIVE

BUT TO DRAW EACH BREATH AT ITS DEEPEST
ITS SWEETEST
AND LIVE.

ANGELA PORTER
LOS ANGELES, CA

QUOTE SOURCES

p. xv   Audre Lorde, "The Transformation of Silence into Language and Action," *Sister Outsider*, Crossing Press, Berkeley, California: 1984.

p. xv   James Baldwin, Quote.

p. 21   Howard Thurman, *Meditations of the Heart*, Beacon Press, Boston: August 1999.

p. 45   Benjamin Mays, "I Knew Carter G. Woodson," *Negro History Bulletin*, Association for the Study of African-American Life and History, Washington, DC.

pg. 57   Ben Carson, Interview, *Good Morning America*, *WABC TV*, NY, NY: November 2002.

p. 69   Colin Powell, Interview, *Nightline*, *WABC TV*, NY, NY: January 2004.

p. 69   Diahann Carroll, Interview By Mike Falcon, *USA Today*, McClean, VA, July 2001.

p. 87 Rev. Martin Luther King Jr., "I Have a Dream," August 1963.

p. 105 Howard Thurman, *Meditations of the Heart*, Beacon Press, Boston: August 1999.

p. 105 Coleman Young, Interview By Ed Gordon, Detroit Free Press, Michigan: April 1988.

p. 119 June Jordan, *Some of Us Did Not Die*, Basic/Civitas, NY, NY: 2002.

p. 135 Audre Lorde, "A Song for Many Moments," *The Black Unicorn*, W.W. Norton & Co., NY, NY: 1978.

Resource Guide

General Cancer Service Organizations

American Cancer Society
1599 Clifton Road NE
Atlanta, GA 30329–4251
(800) ACS-2345
www.cancer.org

The American Cancer Society (ACS) is a nationwide, community-based voluntary health organization. Headquartered in Atlanta, Georgia, the ACS has state divisions and more than 3,400 local offices. The address of a local ACS chapter may be obtained by calling their toll-free telephone number.

Cancer Care
275 7th Avenue
New York, NY 10001
(800) 813–HOPE or (212) 302–2400
www.cancercare.org

A nonprofit organization committed to helping people and their families with cancer. It provides a variety of services, including counseling, education, referrals, publications, and financial assistance.

Cancer Hope Network
2 North Road, Suite A
Chester, NJ 07930
877 HopeNet (Toll Free)
Phone (908) 879–4039
Fax (908) 879–6518
www.Cancerhopenetwork.org

Offers free individualized support to cancer patients currently undergoing treatment.

Cancervive
6500 Wilshire Boulevard, Suite 500
Los Angeles, CA 90048
(310) 203–9232
www.jewishjournal.com

Helps cancer survivors face and overcome the challenges of survivorship.

Coping With Cancer Magazine
P.O. Box 682268
Franklin, TN 37068
Phone (615) 790–2400
Fax (615) 794–0179
www.copingmag.com

America's consumer magazine for people whose lives have been touched by cancer. Provides knowledge, hope and inspiration from cancer survivors and healthcare professionals. Now in its 18th year of service, Coping provides official annual coverage of National Cancer Survivors Day.

National Cancer Institute (NCI)
Cancer Information Service
Building 31, Room 10A16
9000 Rockville Pike
Bethesda, MD 20892
(800) 4–CANCER
www.cancernet.nci.nih.gov

Through CANCERFAX, NCI provides a nationwide telephone service for people with cancer (301) 402–5874. NCI's CANCERFAX provides treatment guidelines, with current data on prognosis, staging, and histological classifications.

NCI's Office of Cancer Survivorship funds research on survivorship issues. NCI's PDQ (Physician Data Query) is the National Cancer Institute's computerized listing of accurate and up-to-date information for patients and health professionals. PDQ also provides information on the latest cancer treatments, research studies, and clinical trials.

National Coalition for Cancer Survivorship
1010 Wayne Avenue
Silver Spring, MD 20910
(301) 650–8868
www.cansearch.org

Organization that addresses the needs of long-term cancer survivors, and advocates for changes in healthcare to maximize survivors' access to optimal treatment and support.

OncoChat
www.oncochat.org

Online peer support for cancer survivors, families and friends.

Wellness Community
919 Eighteenth Street NW, Suite 54

Washington, DC 20006
Phone (202) 659–9709
Fax (202) 659–9301
Toll Free (888) 793–WELL
www.la.wellnesscommunity.org

The Wellness Community provides psychological and emotional support to cancer survivors and their families, free of charge, as an integral part of their medical care.

RESOURCES FOR AFRICAN AMERICANS

Intercultural Cancer Council
6655 Travis, Suite 322
Houston, TX 77030–1312
(713) 798–4617
www.iccnetwork.org

Promotes policies, programs, partnerships, and research to eliminate the unequal burden of cancer among racial and ethnic minorities and medically underserved populations.

National Black Leadership Initiative on Cancer
75 Piedmont Avenue, Suite 450
Atlanta, GA 30303
Office Address
720 Westview Drive
Atlanta, GA 30303
(404) 756–5205
(800) 724–1185
www.nblic.org

A national community outreach program whose principal aim is to positively influence the knowledge and behaviors of African Americans about cancer by providing information in a culturally sensitive manner, and ultimately, to close the cancer racial gap.

National Medical Association
1012 Tenth Street, NW
Washington, D.C. 20001
(202) 347–1895
www.nmanet.org

Promotes the interests of physicians and patients of African descent. Promotes parity in medicine and elimination of health disparities for people of African descent and underserved populations.

AFRICAN-AMERICAN SUPPORT GROUPS AND ORGANIZATIONS AFFILIATED WITH SURVIVORS IN THIS BOOK

Black Cancer Network
P.O. Box 2272
El Segundo, CA 90245
www.blackcancernetwork.org

An online information service for African-American cancer survivors and their families. Provides information about African-American support groups and raises awareness of prevention, early detection, and early diagnosis through education and information.

Breast Cancer Resource Committee
2005 Belmont St. NW
Washington, DC 20009
Phone (202) 463–8040

Fax (202) 463–8015

www.aframerica.com/bcrc

BCRC's mission is to reduce the incidence and mortality rate of breast cancer among African-American women. Services include advocating mammography screening for African-American women aged 35 and older; promoting and reinforcing early detection and treatment of breast cancer through local, national and international outreach; increasing the participation of African-American women in early detection and screening for breast cancer; establishing support groups for African-American women who are survivors of breast cancer; and more.

The Denise Roberts Foundation-Minority Women Fighting Breast Cancer

Centinela Medical Center Fox Hills

6201 Bristol Parkway

Culver City, CA 90230

(888) 8Denise

www.thedeniserobertsfoundation.org

The Denise Roberts Foundation offers minority women low-cost mammograms. Most insurances accepted, referrals to related health care services, educational materials, a videotape series entitled, "Tomorrow: Stories of Survivors," and support groups for cancer survivors and their families.

Sisters Network, Inc.

National Headquarters

8787 Woodway Drive, Suite 4206

Houston, TX 77063–2344

(713) 781–0255; 1 (866) 781–1808

www.sistersnetworkinc.org

A National African-American breast cancer survivorship organization and support group committed to increasing local and national attention on the devastating impact that breast cancer has on the African-American community. Provides contact information on local chapters in 21 states.

These Three Words
10390 Santa Monica Blvd, Fourth Floor
Los Angeles, CA 90025–5058
Phone/Fax (323) 299–3086

A support organization established to benefit the families of terminally ill children at children's hospital in Los Angeles, CA.

For additional information on African-American support organizations, go to Black Cancer Network at www.blackcancernetwork.org.

BOOKS—AFRICAN AMERICANS AND CANCER

Managing Cancer: The African-American's Guide to Prevention, Diagnosis and Treatment
By George Rawls, M.D. & Frank Lloyd, Jr., M.D.
Publisher: Chicago, IL: Hilton Publishing Company
May 2001

Aimed at the specific needs of African Americans, this book is both a complete medical guide and a human exploration of the emotional aspects of cancer. Topics include the prevention, diagnosis and treatment of over twenty types of cancer; how to work with the healthcare system, and the importance of both diet and faith to treatment. Personal stories illustrate the human aspects of the disease, including the joy of successful treatment and the distress when the outcome is death.

That Black Men Might Live: My Fight Against Prostate Cancer
By Reverend Charles Williams, Vernon A. Williams
Publisher: Chicago, IL: Hilton Publishing Company
November 2003

Through the personal story of Reverend Charles Williams, this book addresses the important but often neglected issue of Black men and prostate cancer. More than a biography, this book discusses why and how Black men can break the cycle of health care illiteracy to become aware of their own needs and use the health system to their own benefit. Black men are encouraged to get early and regular physical exams and are guided through what to expect and what to do if they are diagnosed with prostate cancer.

Fine Black Lines: Reflections on Facing Cancer, Fear and Loneliness
By Lois Tschetter Hjelmstad
Publisher: Mulberry Hill Press
May 2003

Thousands have found laughter, tears and realistic optimism as Hjelmstad pulls readers into the deep range of emotions that engulfed her as she battled breast cancer, two mastectomies, and chronic fatigue syndrome. The introspective journal entries, poignant photographs, powerful poetry and thoughtful reflections tell a story that you won't soon forget.

Breast Cancer–Black Women
By Edwin T. Johnson
Publisher: Van Slyke & Bray; 2nd edition
June 2000

This book is dedicated to helping African-American women survive breast cancer by providing valuable information needed to increase early detection and diagnosis.

Cancer! The Day Time Stood Still: An American with African Descent Brown Eyes View
By Antoinette Greene
Publisher: 1st Books Library
April 2003

This book is a personal account of the author's diagnosis of cancer. The author details various emotions, doctor visits, surgeries, complications from treatments and support from family and friends, her medical team and strangers. The book also describes the author's spiritual development in the process of coping with cancer.

Coping: A Black Cancer Patient's Observation
By Warren G. H. Fisher, Jr.
Publisher: iUniverse.com
ISBN: 0595135439, 196 pages
October 2000

Coping is an intriguing story of a Black cancer patient's life experiences. This book is unique because it gives a Black man's view of what he must endure and draw on to recover from something as severe as a cancer bone marrow transplant, and the war that he must fight, not just with himself, but also with those around him.

The Cancer Chronicles
By Audre Lorde
Publisher: Aunt Lute Books
ISBN: 1879960265, 77 pages
October 1980

First published in 1980, this new edition brings together posthumous tributes to Lorde from such writers and poets as Margaret Randall, Jewelle Gomez and Barbara Smith, among others. Using the journal, memoir and essay forms, Lorde gives voice to her feelings and thoughts about the travesty of prosthesis, the pain of amputation, the function of cancer in a profit economy, confrontation with mortality, the strength of women loving, and the power and rewards of self-conscious living.

Celebrating Life: African American Women Speak Out About Breast Cancer
By Sylvania Dunnavant, Sharon Eglebor (editor), Cesar Hallmark (illustrator)
Publisher: USFI Publisher

ISBN: 0964321149, 255 pages
November 1995

This book presents the personal stories of African-American breast cancer survivors. It encourages women to be proactive through the presentation of the experiences of real women (and one man) from varying walks of life.

ADDITIONAL RESOURCES
FOR CANCER SURVIVORS

Resources for Children and Families

American Society of Pediatric Hematology/Oncology (ASPHO)
(847) 375–4716
www.aspho.org

A professional society of Pediatric Hematologists/Oncologists who study and treat childhood cancer and blood disorders.

Candlelighters Childhood Cancer Foundation
3910 Warner Street
Kensington, MD 20895
(800) 366–CCCF or (301) 962–3520
www.candlelighters.org

Provides information, support and advocacy for families of children with cancer and the professionals who care for them.

Childhood Cancer Ombudsman Program
PO Box 595
Burgess, VA 22432
Fax (804) 580–2502 or 2304
Kensington, MD 20895–0498

Phone (800) 366–CCCF
www.candlelighters.org

Outside review by experts in medicine, disability rights, insurance, and employment.

Kids Cancer Network
P.O. Box 4545
Santa Barbara, CA 93140
www.kidscancerrnetwork.org

The Web site contains a bimonthly FUNLETTER magazine (also available in Spanish), a resource center, Affection Connection appreciation certificates for medical caregivers, pen-friend program, prayer network, and "your story" sharing area.

Kids Konnected
27071 Cabot Road, Suite 102
Laguna Hills, CA 92653
(800) 899–2866, (949) 582–5443
www.kidskonnected.org

Provides friendship, education, and support to kids who have a parent with cancer.

Locks of Love
2925 10th Avenue North, Suite 102
Lake Worth, FL 33401
Phone (561) 963–1677
Fax (561) 963–9914
Toll Free (888) 896–1588

A nonprofit organization that provides hairpieces to financially disadvantaged children under the age of 18 suffering from long-term hair loss.

Make-a-Wish Foundation of America
3550 North Central Avenue, Suite 300
Phoenix, AZ 85012–2127
1 (800) 722–WISH (9474)
www.wish.org

The mission is to grant the wishes of children with life threatening conditions.

The Miracle Kids
www.themiraclekids.com

Kids and their stories as told by their families

Make a Child Smile
www.makeachildsmile.org

Stories of courageous kids with life-threatening illnesses. Supporters are asked to mail a nice card or small gift to the featured kids of the month.

National Childhood Cancer Foundation
440 E. Huntington Dr.
P.O. Box 60012
Arcadia, CA 91066–6012
(800) 458–6223
www.NCCF.org

Supports the research and treatment programs of the Children's Oncology Group at over 235 member-institutions in North America and abroad. Also advocates for children with cancer and their families.

Pediatric Oncology Resource Center
www.acor.org/ped-onc

One stop center for parents of children with cancer by parents of children with cancer.

Ronald McDonald House
Ronald McDonald House Charities
One Kroc Drive
Oak Brook, IL 60523
Phone (630) 623–7048
Fax (630) 623–7488
www.rmhc.com

Offers a refuge from the hospital, a "home-away-from-home."

Governmental Agencies

Centers for Disease Control & Prevention
Office of Minority Health
Mailstop E-67
1600 Clifton Road, NE
Atlanta, Georgia 30333
(404) 498–2320
www.cdc.gov.omh

Mission is to eliminate racial and ethnic health care disparities.

National Health Information Center
(A service of the U.S. Dept. of Health and Human Services—
Office of Disease Prevention and Health Promotion)
(800) 336–4797
Rockville, Maryland
www.nhic-nt.health.org

Health information resources in the federal government.

US Public Health Service's Office on Women's Health
Hot line (800) 994–9662, TDD (888) 220–5446
www.4women.gov

Resource center for the nation's 10 million disabled women. Offers information on disabilities, laws, statistics, access to healthcare, financial assistance, abuse, parenting, sexuality, and links to advocacy groups.

Employment/Disability Information

Equal Employment Opportunity Commission
1801 L Street NW
Washington, DC 20507
(800) 669–4000
www.eeoc.gov/mediate

Provides information on how to enforce your rights under the Americans with Disabilities Act.

National Rehabilitation Information Center
4200 Forbes Blvd., Suite 20
Lanham, MD 20706-4829
(800) 346–2742
www.naric.com

Federally funded information service collects and distributes books, journal articles, and audiovisuals concerning disability and rehabilitation.

U.S. Department of Justice Civil Rights Division
Disability Rights Section
950 Pennsylvania Avenue NW
Washington, DC 20530
(800) 514–0301, TDD (800) 514–0383
www.usdoj.gov

Specialists answer questions about Title I and Title II of the Americans with Disabilities Act.

U.S. Department of Labor
Employment Standards Division
Frances Perkins Building
200 Constitution Avenue, NW
Washington, D.C. 20210
1–866–4–USWAGE
www.dol.gov/esa/whd/fmla

Provides information on the Family Medical Leave Act.

American Council on Education–HEATH Resource Center
One Dupont Circle NW
Washington, DC 20036
(800) 544–3284
www.heath-resource-center.org

HEATH is the national clearinghouse on post-secondary education for individuals with disabilities. It provides information about educational support services, policies, procedures, adaptations, and opportunities at American campuses and vocational-technical schools.

The Disability Rights Education and Defense Fund
2212 Sixth Street
Berkeley, CA 94710
(800) 466–4232 or (510) 644–2555
www.dredf.org

Answers questions about the Americans with Disabilities Act and explains how to file a complaint.

Job Accommodation Network (JAN)
West Virginia University
P.O. Box 6080
Morgantown, WV 26506

(800) 526–7234 or (800) ADA-WORK

www.jan.wvu.edu

An international consulting service that provides free information about how employers can accommodate people with disabilities. The service also provides information on the Americans with Disabilities Act (ADA).

National Association of Protection and Advocacy Systems
900 2nd Street NE, Suite 211
Washington, DC 20002
(202) 408–9514

www.napas.org

For help with Social Security income, disability rights issues, or violations of special education law.

National Employment Lawyer's Association
44 Montgomery Street, Suite 2080
San Francisco, CA 94107
Phone (415) 256–7629
Fax (415) 677–9445

www.nela.org

A non-profit, professional organization of more than 3,400 lawyers who represent individual employees in cases involving employment discrimination, wrongful termination, employee benefits, and other employment-related matters.

Patient Advocate Foundation
700 Thimble Shales Boulevard, Suite 200
Newport News, VA 23606
(800) 532–5274 or (757) 873–8999

www.patientadvocate.org

Serves as an active liaison between the patient and the insurer, employer and/or creditors to resolve insurance, job retention and or debt crisis matters.

Medical Insurance

Association of Community Cancer Centers
Reimbursement Hotlines
11600 Nebel Street, Suite 201
Rockville, MD 20852–2557
Phone (301) 984–9496
Fax (301) 770–1949
www.accc-cancer.org/publications/hotlines.asp

Provides a yearly listing of reimbursement assistance programs for oncology-related services.

Healthinsuranceinfo.net
Health Policy Institute
Attn: Consumer Guides
2233 Wisconsin Avenue, NW
Suite 525
Washington, DC 20007
www.healthinsuranceinfo.net

Provides a consumer guide for getting and keeping health insurance in every state and District of Columbia.

Types of Cancer

Brain Tumor

American Brain Tumor Association
2720 River Road, Suite 146
Des Plaines, IL 60018
Phone (800) 886–2282

Fax (847) 827–9918

www.abta.org

Offers free publications, educational programs and lists of physicians and other resources.

The Brain Tumor Society
124 Watertown Street, Suite 3–H
Watertown, MA 02472
(800) 770–8287
(617) 924–9997
www.tbts.org

Provides individualized patient/family information, publishes educational material, sponsors professional and patient conferences, and funds research.

Children's Brain Tumor Foundation
274 Madison Avenue, Suite 1301
New York, NY 10016
Phone (866) 228–4673, (212) 448–9494
Fax (212) 448–1022
www.cbtf.org

Offers a free resource guide (in English and Spanish), the Parent-To-Parent Network, telephone support groups, newsletter and an annual teleconference and funds research.

National Brain Tumor Foundation
22 Battery Street, Suite 612
San Francisco, CA 94111–5520
Phone (800) 934–2873, (510) 839–9777
Fax (510) 839–9779
www. braintumor.org

Offers contact with other brain tumor patients, information about treatment and local conferences, a listing of support groups, and a newsletter. Raises funds for brain tumor research.

Pediatric Brain Tumor Foundation
302 Ridgefield Court
Ashville, NC 28806
Phone (800) 253–6530
Fax (828) 665–6894
www.pbtfus.org

Funds medical research grants to help find the cause and cure of childhood brain tumors. Offers support programs for families of a child with a brain tumor. Services include free literature, a newsletter, and an internet conference series.

Breast Cancer

National Breast Cancer Coalition
1101 Seventeenth Street, NW, Suite 1300
Washington, DC 20036
www.natbcc.org

Formed to eradicate breast cancer through action and advocacy. Main goals include research, advocacy for access to treatment and influence public policy.

Susan G. Komen Breast Cancer Foundation
5005 LBJ Freeway, Suite 250
Dallas, TX 75244
Phone (800) 462–9273
Fax (972) 855–1605 (fax)
www.komen.org.

Dedicated to eradicating breast cancer as a life-threatening disease by advancing research, education, screening and treatment. Annually awards research grants and fellowships.

Women's Information Network (WIN) Against Breast Cancer
536 S. Second Avenue, Suite K
Covina, CA 91723–3043
1 (866) 294–6222
www.winabc.org

Mission is to increase public awareness about breast cancer and ensure that individuals from all socioeconomic backgrounds have rapid access to current and relevant education, support and information about this disease.

Y-Me National Breast Cancer Organization
212 W. Van Buren, Suite 1000
Chicago, IL 60607
(800) 221–2141 (24 hour hotline with interpreters in 150 languages)
(800) 986–9505 (24 hour Spanish)
www.y-me.org

Provides peer counseling on a 24–hour hotline. Breast health and breast cancer resource in ten affiliate communities in the U.S. through peer support, educational programs, local resources and advocacy initiatives. Offers educational workshops, wig and prosthesis banks and support groups.

Colon Cancer

Colon Cancer Alliance
175 9th Avenue
New York, NY 10011
Phone (877) 422–2030, (212) 627–7451

Fax (425) 947–6147

www.ccalliance.org

Organization made up of survivors and caregivers. Services include a buddy program, educational materials, clinical trial information, and news about colorectal cancer treatment and research.

Colorectal Cancer Network

P.O. Box 182

Kensington, MD 20895–0182

(301) 879–1500

www.colorectal-cancer.net

Website has extensive information on colon, rectal, anal and appendiceal cancers. Provides free resource packet for newly diagnosed; education; connection to other survivors.

Gastric/Stomach Cancer

See the American Cancer Society or the National Cancer Institute for information.

Gynecologic Cancers

Gilda's Club Worldwide

322 Eighth Avenue, Suite 1402

New York, NY 10001

Phone (888) GILDA-4–U, (917) 305–1200

Fax (917) 305–0549

www.gildasclub.org

International network where men, women and children with cancer and their families and friends join with others to build social and emotional support as a supplement to medical care in a free, nonresidential, home-like

*setting. People with all kinds and stages of cancer are welcome in 16
locations open worldwide.*

Gynecologic Cancer Foundation
401 N. Michigan Avenue
Chicago, IL 60611
Phone (800) 444–4441, (312) 644–6610
Fax (312) 527–6658
www.wcn.org/gct

*Designed to increase public awareness of ways to prevent, detect and treat
gynecological cancers and supports innovative research.*

Ovarian Cancer National Alliance
910 17th Street NW, Suite 413
Washington, DC 20006
(202) 331–1332
www.ovariancancer.org

*A consumer-led umbrella organization uniting ovarian cancer survivors,
women's health activists and healthcare professionals in a coordinated effort
to focus national attention on ovarian cancer.*

The Ovarian Cancer Research Fund
14 Pennsylvania Plaza, Suite 1400
New York, NY 10122
Phone (800) 873–9569
Fax (212) 947–5652
www. ocrt.org

*Dedicated to advancing research by underwriting investigations to find
techniques for early detection and to aid in the development of new
therapies. Raises awareness through educational outreach programs, and
awareness projects, including videos and resource materials.*

National Ovarian Cancer Coalition
500 NE Spanish River Blvd., Suite 14
Boca Baton, FL 33431
Phone (888) OVARIAN, (561) 393–0005
Fax (561) 393–7275
www.ovarian.org

Raises awareness to promote early detection and education about the disease. Sponsors education seminars for healthcare providers and educational forums for the public.

Kidney Cancer

Kidney Cancer Association
1234 Sherman Avenue, Suite 203
Evanston, IL 60202–1375
Phone (800) 850–9132
Fax (847) 332–2978
www.kidneycancerassociation.org

Dedicated to finding a cure for kidney cancer; increasing funding for research; getting new drugs tried and approved; and supporting patients.

Leukemia/Lymphoma/Myeloma/Sarcoma

The Leukemia & Lymphoma Society
1311 Mamaroneck Avenue
White Plains, NY 10605
Info Resource Center (800) 955–4572
General Information (914) 949–5213
Fax (914) 821–3607
www.leukemia-lymphoma.org

Dedicated to seeking the cause and eventual cure of leukemia, lymphoma and myeloma. Programs include research funding, patient aid, peer support, family support groups and education.

Lymphoma Research Foundation
111 Broadway, 19th Floor
New York, NY 10005
(212) 349–2910; (800) 235–6848
www.lymphoma.org

The mission is to eradicate lymphoma and serve those touched by the disease.

International Myeloma Foundation
12650 Riverside Drive, Suite 206
N. Hollywood, CA 91607
Phone (800) 452–CURE, (818) 487–7455
Fax (818) 487–7454
www. myelcma.org

Dedicated to improving the quality of life of myeloma patients while working toward prevention and a cure. Operates a Myeloma Hotline, disseminates information, on the best seminars and workshops for the patient community and medical professionals, and funds research.

Multiple Myeloma Research Foundation
3 Forest Street
New Canaan, CT 06840
Phone (203) 972–1250
Fax (203) 972–1259
www. multiplemyeloma.org

Supports research grants and professional symposia on multiple myeloma. Publishes a quarterly newsletter, conducts seminars, and provides referrals and information packets.

The Sarcoma Alliance
775 E. Blithedale Ave., #334
Mill Valley, CA 94941
Phone (415) 381–7236
Fax (415) 381–7235
www.sarcomaalliance.org

Provides education and support to sarcoma patients and their families, friends and caregivers.

Lung Cancer

Alliance for Lung Cancer Advocacy, Support and Education
888 16th St. NW, Suite 800
Washington, DC 20006
www.alcase.org
Phone (202) 463–2080
Toll Free (800) 298–2436

Provides support to people at risk for and living with lung cancer.

American Lung Association
61 Broadway, 6th Floor,
New York, NY 10006–2701
(212) 315–8700
www.lungusa.org

Dedicated to preventing lung disease and promoting lung health.

Oral, Head and Neck

Support for People with Oral and Head and Neck Cancer
(SPOHNC)
PO Box 53

Locust Valley, NY 11560–0053
(516) 759–5333
www.spohnc.org

Nonprofit organization dedicated to meeting the needs of oral, head and neck cancer survivors.

International Association of Laryngectomees
P.O. Box 691060
Stockton, CA 95269–1060
Phone (866) 425–3678
Fax (209) 472–0516
www.larynxlink.com

An association of over 200 laryngectomees' clubs. Clubs provide pre- and post-operation visits to laryngeal cancer patients and continuing support and education for laryngectomees and families.

Pancreatic Cancer

Pancreatic Cancer Action Network
2221 Rosecrans Ave., Suite 131
El Segundo, CA 90245
Phone (877) 272–6226
Fax (310) 725–0029
www.pancan.org

Works to focus national attention on the need to find the cure for pancreatic cancer by providing advocacy, awareness and education to patients and professionals.

Prostate Cancer and Urological Disease

American Foundation for Urologic Disease
1000 Corporate Blvd, Suite 410
Linthicum, MD 21090
(800) 828–7866
(410) 689–3990
(410) 689–3998
www.afud.org

Dedicated to the prevention and cure of urologic diseases through the expansion of research, education, awareness and advocacy programs.

National Prostate Cancer Coalition
1154 15th Street NW
Washington, DC 20005
Phone (202) 463–9455
Fax (202) 463–9456
E-mail: info@pcacoalition.org
www.pcacoalition.org

A grassroots advocacy organization seeking to increase prostate cancer awareness and enhance outreach; advocates for research funds and better detection strategies.

Skin Cancer

The Skin Cancer Foundation
PO Box 561
New York, NY 10156
800–SKIN-490
www.skincancer.org

Conducts education programs and supports research to reduce the incidence, morbidity and mortality of the disease. Educational materials available.

Clinical Trials

The National Cancer Institute's PDQ Clinical Trial Database
www.cancer.gov/clinicaltrials
(800) 4–CANCER

Contains information on over 1700 open clinical trials, mostly in the U.S.

Coalition of National Cancer Cooperative Groups
1818 Market Street, #1100
Philadelphia, PA 19103
(877) 520–4457
www.CancerTrialsHelp.org

Web site contains "Trial Check," cancer clinical trials search engine, and an interactive training guide, "Cancer Research: A Guide to Cancer Clinical Trials."

Radiation Oncology Therapy Group (RTOG) Trials
1101 Market Street, 14th Floor
Philadelphia, PA 19107
Toll Free (800) 227–5463, ext. 4189
Phone (215) 574–3189
Fax (215) 923–1737
www.rtog.org
www.411cancer.com

Offers a clinical trials database that is a useful database of industry sponsored cancer trials. A cancer cooperative research group focusing on radiation therapy. All of the RTOG trials are in the NCI's PDQ database, however what distinguishes RTOG's offering is that they make the complete protocol document for every RTOG trial freely available to everyone.

Phrma
1100 Fifteenth Street, NW
Washington, DC 20005

Phone (202) 835–3400
Fax (202) 835–3414
www.phrma.org

An American pharmaceutical industry trade group with some important information on drugs in development. The Phrma New Medicines in Development Database is a rather comprehensive list of drugs in clinical testing which can be queried by disease.

Bone Marrow Transplant Information

Blood & Marrow Transplant Information Network
2310 Skokie Valley Road, Suite 104
Highland Park, IL 60035
Toll Free (888) 597–7674
Phone (847) 433–3313
Fax (847) 433–4599
www.bmtinfonet.org

Links transplant patients with survivors, maintains a directory of transplant centers and helps with insurance problems.

Blood and Marrow Transplant Clinical Trials Network
401 N. Washington St.
Suite 700
Rockville, MD 20850
www.bmtctn.net
E-mail: bmtctn@emmes.com

Conducts large multi-institutional clinical trials to address important issues in hematopoietic stem cell transplantation (HSCT). Designed to maintain continuity of transplant centers and centers with collaborators at the National Institute of Health, and to offer trial participation to patients in all regions of the U.S.

Bonemarrowtest.com
1(800) 915–3695
www.bonemarrowtest.com

Provides HLA testing services to the NMDP and other registries, as well as to individual donors who do not wish to join a public registry.

Caitlin Raymond International Registry
University of Massachusetts Medical Center
55 Lake Ave. N.
Worcester, MA 01655
(800) 726–2824
E-mail: info@crir.org
www.crir.org

A donor registry for patients and physicians conducting searches for unrelated bone marrow donors or cord blood units.

Cancer Links
Bone Marrow Transplants
E-mail: marriage@seidata.com
www.seidata.com/~marriage/rcancer.html#bmt

Links to information on bone marrow transplants.

National Bone Marrow Transplant Link
20411 W. 12 Mile Road
Suite 108
Southfield, MI 48076
(800) 546–5268
E-mail: nbmtlink@aol.com
www.nbmtlink.org

Provides resources and support to potential bone marrow transplant patients and their families.

National Marrow Donor Program
3001 Broadway Street NE, Suite 500
Minneapolis, MN 55413
Phone (800) MARROW 2
Fax (612) 627–5877
Office of Patient Advocacy
(888) 999–6743
www.marrow.org.

Facilitates unrelated blood stem cell transplants and maintains a registry of nearly five million volunteer donors, offers matching services and patient services and conducts research.

Infertility

National Infertility Network Exchange
PO Box 204
East Meadow, NY 11554
(516) 794–5772
www.nine-infertility.org

Nonprofit organization that offers peer support for infertile couples, referral to appropriate professionals, and educational materials.

Fertile Hope
PO Box 624
New York, NY 10014
Phone (888) 994–HOPE
Fax (212) 202–3692
www.fertilehope.org

Provides reproductive information, support and hope to cancer survivors whose medical treatments present the risk of infertility.

Home Health Care/Hospice Care

Growth House, Inc.

(415) 863–3045

www.growthhouse.org

Provides resources for life-threatening illness and end of life care to improve the quality of compassionate care for people who are dying. Provides access to the most comprehensive collection of reviewed resources for palliative and end of life care.

The National Hospice and Palliative Care Organization (NHPCO)

1700 Diagonal Road

Suite 625

Alexandria, VA 22314

(703) 837–1500

(800) 658–8898 (Helpline)

E-mail: info@nhpco.org

www.nhpco.org

An association of programs that provide hospice and palliative care. Provides information about how to find a hospice and about the financial aspects of hospice.

The Hospice Association of America

228 Seventh Street, SE

Washington, DC 20003

(202) 546–4759

Provides facts and statistics about hospice programs and can also supply the publication "Information About Hospice: A Consumer's Guide."

Physician Select Program

American Medical Association
515 N. State Street
Chicago, IL 60610
(800) 621–8335

AMA physicians select provides primary source-verified information on all U.S. licensed physicians from which consumers can select a physician or verify the credentials of a known physician. This means that all data have been verified for accuracy and authenticated by accrediting agencies, medical schools, residency training programs, licensing and certifying boards, and other date sources.

Other Resources

Corporate Angel Network, Inc.
One Loop Road, Westchester County Airport
White Plains, NY 10604-1215
Patient Care (866) 328–1313
General Phone (914) 328–1313
Fax (914) 328–3938
www.corpangelnetwork.org

Arranges free air transportation for cancer patients and bone marrow donors to/from cancer treatment centers nationwide. There are no financial requirements or limits on the number of flights. Patients must be able to walk and travel without life support.

Inquiries About Physicians

American Board of Medical Specialties
1007 Church Street, Suite 404
Evanston, Illinois 60201-5913
Phone Verification (866) ASK–ABMS
Phone (847) 491–9091
Fax (847) 328–3596

A not-for-profit organization that oversees physician certification in the U.S. Also helps to improve the quality of medical care.

Note: There are many more resources available to support cancer patients. For additional information, contact you local American Cancer Society office or contact your doctor.